Aromatherapy

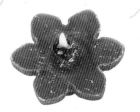

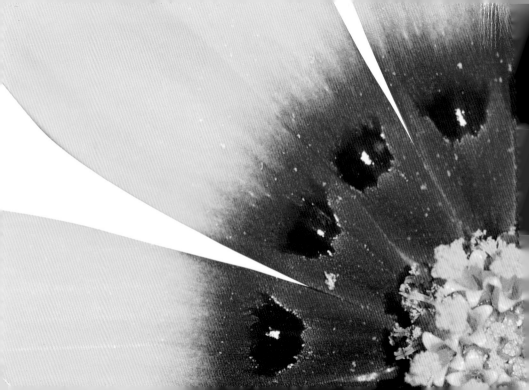

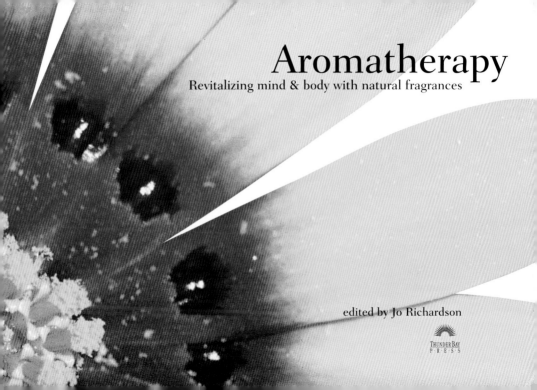

Aromatherapy

Revitalizing mind & body with natural fragrances

edited by Jo Richardson

THUNDER BAY
P·R·E·S·S

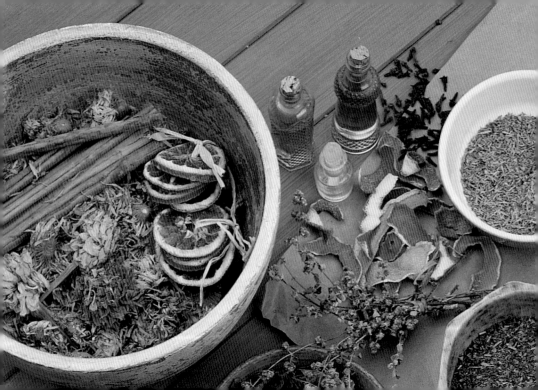

MANAGING EDITOR Simon Tuite
PROJECT EDITOR Jo Richardson
DESIGNER Louise Clements
PRODUCTION Neil Randles; Karen Staff

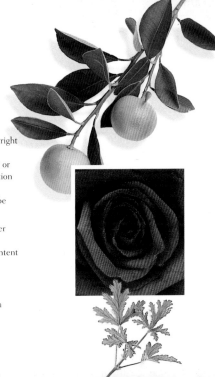

Published in the United States by Thunder Bay Press
An imprint of the Advantage Publishers Group
5880 Oberlin Drive, San Diego, CA 92121-4794
www.advantagebooksonline.com
Copyright © Salamander Books Limited, 2001
A member of the Chrysalis Group plc

All notations of errors or omissions should be addressed to Thunder
Bay Press, editorial department, at the above address. All other
correspondence (author inquiries, permissions) concerning the content
of this book should be addressed to Salamander Books Limited, 8
Blenheim Court, Brewery Road, London N7 9NY, England.

ISBN 1-57145-567-1
Library of Congress Cataloging-in-Publication Data available upon
request.

Produced by Toppan
Printed in China

1 2 3 4 5 01 02 03 04

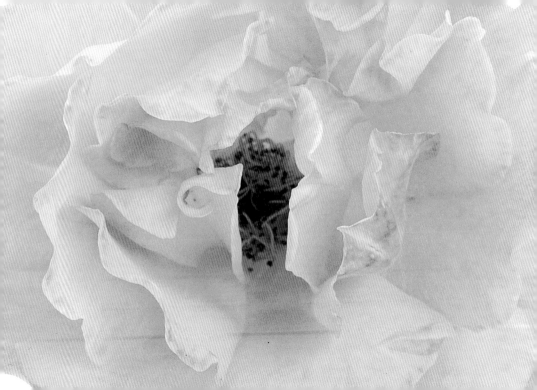

contents

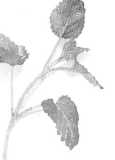

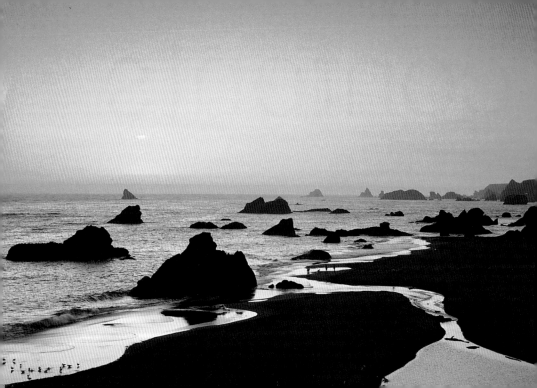

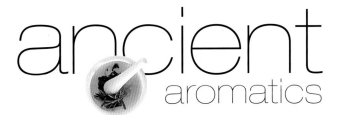

ancient
aromatics

basic instinct

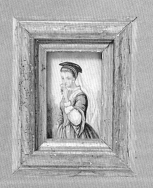

Smell is probably the most basic—and most potent—of all human instincts. Scent is the unseen power that strongly influences our lives, from infancy onward. We often recall personal experiences and important happenings through distinctive scents.

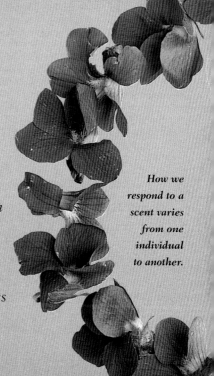

Our neolithic ancestors followed their noses to find food, detect enemies, and track down a mate. Early on in our history, culinary and medicinal herbs became a functional part of daily life, but their aromatic qualities soon became a source of pleasure, too.

How we respond to a scent varies from one individual to another.

soul scents

Scent imprinting was an important part of some early religions, creating an atmosphere of rest and spiritual awareness.

The ancient Egyptians believed that cedarwood was imperishable and able to preserve anyone enclosed in it, and cedar oil was rubbed into bodies and the wood burnt as incense, as an offering to the gods. They also believed that when their prayers mixed with incense smoke, they would ascend to heaven more rapidly.

The Koran, the Holy Scripture for Muslims, describes Paradise as being filled with nymphs created out of musk. The followers of the Prophet Mohammed were so fond

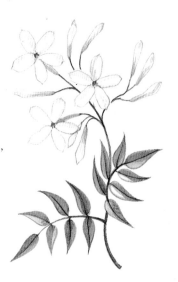

of musk that it was frequently mixed with mortar in the construction of mosques.

In China, about 500 B.C., the philosopher Confucius wrote that temples were hung with blossoms of magnolia, peach, jasmine, and jonquil. Incense was burned in homes as well as mosques. Burning incense was also adopted by the Christian faith and became part of many religious services. This practice continues today in the Catholic church.

early aromatherapy

In addition to using perfumes in religious rites, the ancient Egyptians used them in their toilet preparations and in body massages to increase the elasticity of the skin, which is essential in hot climates where it soon becomes dry and wrinkled. They began to import aromatic plants and potions 2,000 years before the birth of Christ. The Greeks and Romans took up the use of essential oils. Julius Caesar (100–44 B.C.) forbade them since he regarded them as effeminate, but the Roman Emperor Caligula (A.D. 12–41) embraced them with enthusiasm, and their use was popularized in the ever-widening Roman Empire. Crusaders returning to Europe from the Holy Land in the 11th–13th centuries added to their knowledge.

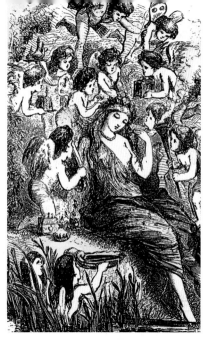

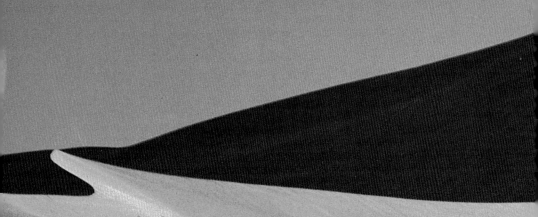

scents of the past Some fragrances have been highly prized since antiquity. Myrrh has always been considered a potent and valuable aromatic. It is reputed that the Queen of Sheba ensnared King Solomon by using oil of myrrh. Such was the value put upon the essence that it was one

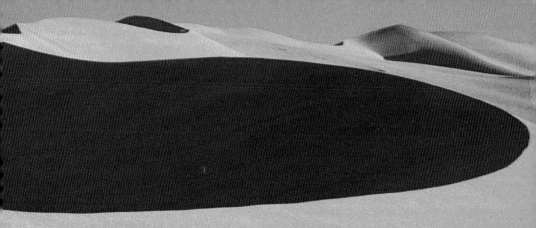

of the precious gifts presented to the infant Jesus by the Three Kings, along with frankincense, a sacred scent widely used by the ancient Egyptians and the Chinese in religious rituals. Both frankincense and myrrh were discovered in Tutankhamun's tomb when it was opened in 1922.

age-old remedies

In the Middle Ages, as successive plagues swept across Europe and the Middle East, physicians and herbalists searched the plant kingdom for cures and preventative measures.

Flowers, fruit, leaves, resins, barks, and herbs that are still well known today played an essential role in the treatment of illness—rosemary, sage, peppermint, oranges, and cloves, for example.

Across the world, our ancestors have sought natural cures for weaknesses of both mind and body. The Maoris in

New Zealand used the plant now called tea tree for bathing cuts, wounds, and burns. Modern science has since revealed it to be a powerful antiseptic.

Native Americans treated skin conditions with an infusion of spruce—now analyzed as being rich in vitamin C.

Herbal medicine was used in ancient China to treat a wide variety of ailments.

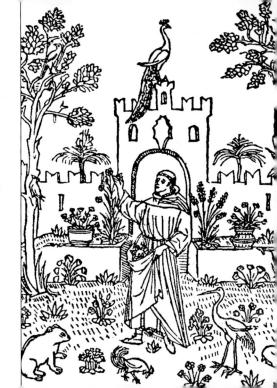

healing scents

During the 16th and 17th centuries, botanists classified plants according to their healing powers. By the 1700s, 13 essential oils had been listed for medicinal use. But as medical science developed, interest in herbal cures diminished.

In the early part of the 1900s, the French chemist René Maurice Gattefossé burned his hand while working in the laboratory of a perfumery. To relieve the pain, he plunged it into the nearest cold liquid which, by happy coincidence, was lavender oil. His hand healed astonishingly quickly with little or no scarring. He was so impressed by this event that he resolved to investigate the medicinal powers of other essential oils.

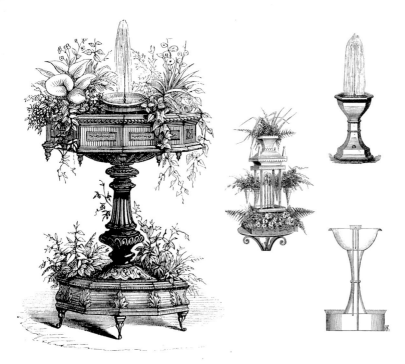

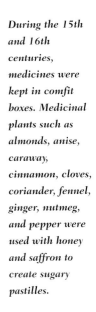

During the 15th and 16th centuries, medicines were kept in comfit boxes. Medicinal plants such as almonds, anise, caraway, cinnamon, cloves, coriander, fennel, ginger, nutmeg, and pepper were used with honey and saffron to create sugary pastilles.

napoleon's flower

Napoleon, like many other people, found the fragrance of violets appealing and memorable. He derived great pleasure and comfort from these delicate flowers, and gave bouquets of them to Josephine on their wedding anniversaries. Ladies who gathered to receive him carried posies of the Emperor's best-loved flower. When banished to Elba, he said: "I will return with the violets in the spring." For this reason, violets became a symbol of Bonapartists, and Napoleon became known as "Père Violette."

After his defeat at Waterloo and before his departure to St. Helena, Napoleon is said to have visited Josephine's grave, where he picked violets, their favorite flower, which he then carefully placed in a locket.

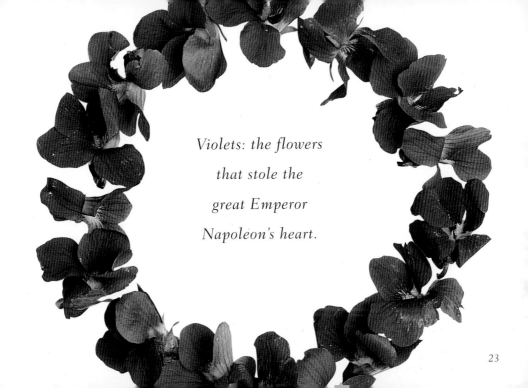

Violets: the flowers that stole the great Emperor Napoleon's heart.

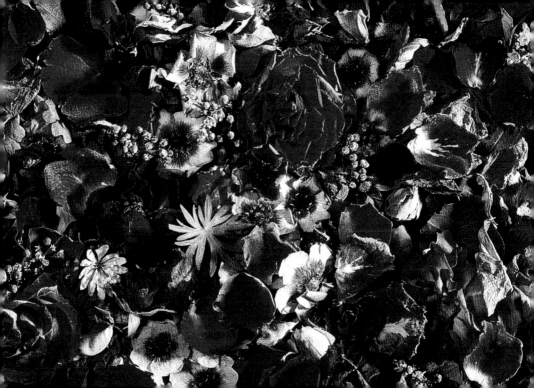

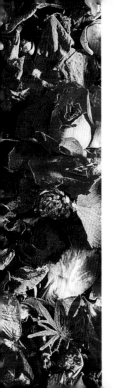

essentials

nature's essences

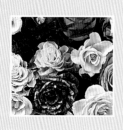

At the heart of aromatherapy are essential oils—
"concentrated smells." No one is completely sure exactly
what they are, although scientists have analyzed many of
their chemical constituents. They are naturally
occurring substances found in tiny sacs in different parts of plants: flowers,
leaves, bark, berries, stems, and roots. Different parts of the same plant may

produce various oils. For example,

petitgrain comes from orange leaves, orange oil

from the peel of the fruit, and neroli from the

blossom. The range of essential oils is wide and at

first glance appears bewildering, but most have familiar common

names and many come from plants commonly found in ordinary gardens.

27

extracting the essence

Extracting essential oils is a complicated process. Many are obtained by distillation. The relevant part of the plant is processed by steam in a vat, and the oil is then separated from the cooled, condensed water. Lavender oil is produced this way. Essential oils from very fragile flowers, such as ylang ylang and jasmine, are obtained by solvent extraction because the heat and pressure of distillation would destroy the oil. Oils extracted by this method are called absolutes—rose absolute, for example. Oils from fruit peel are squeezed into special sponges, barks are usually powdered before distillation, and gums and resins are dissolved in solvents.

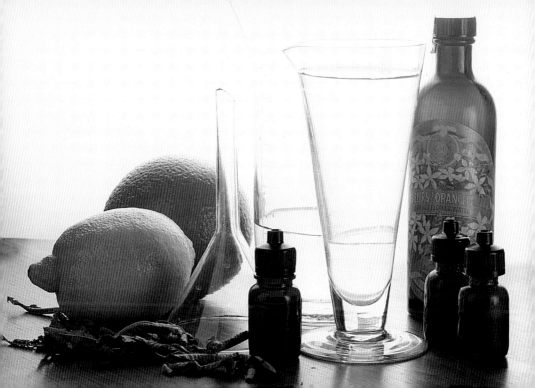

choosing & storing

Essential oils are extremely volatile, but not at all greasy. They are usually supplied in dark glass bottles and should be stored in these bottles in a cool place and out of direct sunlight. Do not use plastic containers because they can be damaged by the oils.

Buy oils from a reputable source to guarantee their purity and quality.

Look for the words "pure essential oil" on the label—synthetic oils and diluted mixtures do not have the same potency. Price varies according to the source of the oil. Many useful oils are fairly inexpensive; others are a luxurious treat—it takes about a ton of rose petals to produce 1 pound of rose oil!

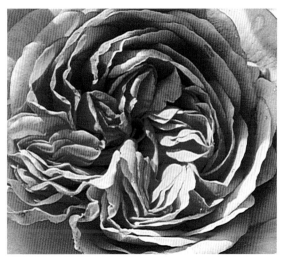

aromagic

There are numerous ways of using essential oils and benefiting from their powerful effects. Massage is the technique mainly used by professional aromatherapists and is the best known and most effective way of using the oils. See Chapter 3, pages 152–213, for advice on how to use oils in massage and for step-by-step massage techniques.

Another very popular way of using essential oils is in a bath. A few drops of pine, neroli, or jasmine oil in a tub of warm or hot water can be energizing, relaxing, or sensuous, depending on the oil you choose. Add a total of 5 drops of your oil, or mixture of oils, to the water and stir. Step in without delay, then lie back and enjoy the experience for at least 15 minutes.

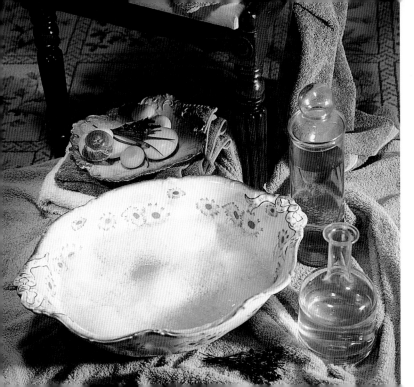

You can also use essential oils as room fragrancers, by using a vaporizer, where the scent is gently dispersed and you are barely aware of breathing it in—see pages 218–221.

33

Essential oils can be used at home to help you soothe away all those minor stresses and strains of everyday life—from a headache to a hangover, from overwork to insomnia, from indigestion to jet lag.

LINDA DOESER: *The Fragrant Art of Aromatherapy* (1995)

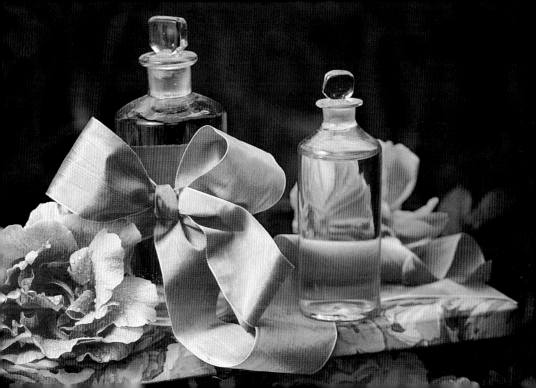

health scents

Direct inhalation is another popular method of using essential oils. When you are suffering from a bad cold or cough, fill a bowl with hot water, add a few drops of the appropriate oil, then cover your head with a towel. Close your eyes and inhale deeply for several minutes. The steam rising from the hot water opens the pores of the skin, so you can use an essential oil this way for a facial. Two or three drops of eucalyptus oil on the pillow at night should provide a snuffle-free rest, while a couple of drops of lavender can help immeasurably in counter-acting insomnia. You can also sprinkle your handkerchief or a tissue with a couple of drops of calming, energizing, or decongestant oil to inhale during the day.

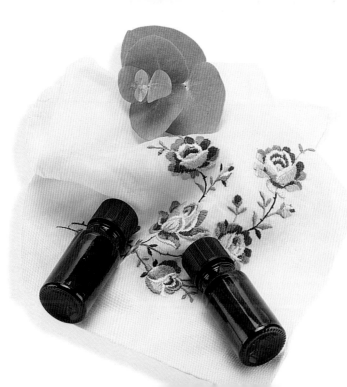

At critical times, you can simply unscrew the top of a bottle of an appropriate essential oil and breathe deeply.

compresses

Cold compresses are an age-old remedy for relieving the pain of bruising, muscular stress, headaches, and rashes, as well as for reducing inflammation and fever. Pour 2 or 3 cups of cold water into a bowl and add 6 ice cubes. Add 5 drops of the appropriate oil, dip in a clean cloth, and ring it out, then place it over the sore area.

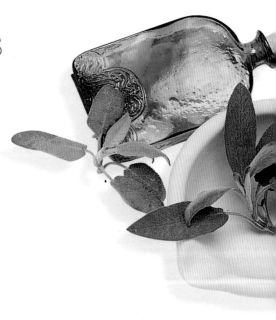

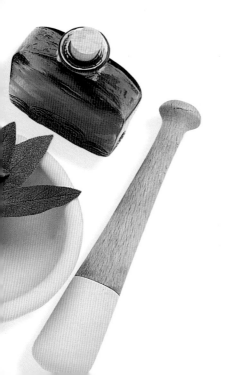

poultices

A hot poultice works in much the same way for relieving muscular pain, earache, backache, stomach ache, sore throat, or congestion due to colds and flu. Pour 2 or 3 cups of very hot water into a bowl and add 5 drops of the appropriate oil. Wear rubber gloves for wringing out the cloth, and make sure it is not scalding hot when you apply it to the skin.

aromacare

Essential oils can also be used in all kinds of beauty preparations, including cleansers, masks, and moisturizers (see pages 262–303). Some are excellent for treating dull and lifeless hair, dandruff and other scalp conditions, and for thinning hair. A little lemon oil can be added to water for a manicure, and you can create a sensuous footbath by adding a few drops of essential oil.

Essential oils are excellent to use around the house, and many of the naturally antiseptic oils make good cleansers. You can add a drop or two of essential oil to garbage cans to keep them clean and sweet-smelling. A couple of drops of oil on a cotton ball can be placed inside the vacuum cleaner bag to scent the air when you are cleaning floors and furniture. Use the deodorizing properties of essential oils by placing a cotton ball with a few drops of oil inside your closet or laundry basket.

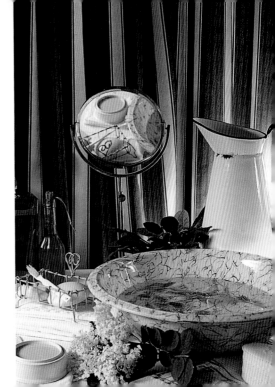

a word of caution

Essential oils are very potent. Never apply them undiluted to skin and do not exceed the stated number of drops. If an oil causes irritation, wash the skin immediately and apply a little almond or other bland oil to the affected area. Symptoms should disappear within an hour, but consult a medical practitioner if not. People with known allergies should consult a qualified aromatherapist before using essential oils.

Treatment of serious illnesses is best left to a qualified aromatherapist, who will take a holistic approach to your condition and who has thorough knowledge of the physical and psychological effects of essential oils.

If you are seeking treatment for a medical condition, consult your regular medical practitioner first.

Oils not recommended for home use:
Cinnamon, clove, hyssop, and sage.

Oils to avoid during pregnancy: Basil, clove, cinnamon, fennel, hyssop, juniper, marjoram, myrrh, peppermint, rosemary, sage, and white thyme.

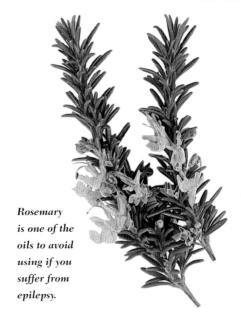

Rosemary is one of the oils to avoid using if you suffer from epilepsy.

safety
for babies & children

Essential oils can be used effectively on babies and children, but dosages should be reduced as specified below. When massaging babies and children, use only your fingertips.

Babies up to one year: Use only lavender oil or chamomile oil. Use only 1 drop of the appropriate oil for a compress, in a warm bath, or in a vaporizer. You can also add 1 drop to 1 tablespoon of carrier oil for a very gentle massage (see pages 152–153).

Ages 1–6: Tea tree oil can be used in addition to lavender and chamomile for children over one year old. Use 1–3 drops in the same way as previously directed.

Ages 7-12: Use half the number of drops recommended for adults.

Ages 12 plus: Use essential oils as directed for adults, but introduce new ones slowly and watch for any adverse reactions.

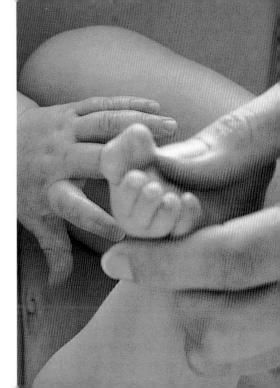

Floral Oils

As well as being extracted
from flowers of plants, together with
the leaves in some cases, these oils
have sweet, flowery scents—some
delicate, others heavy and sensuous.

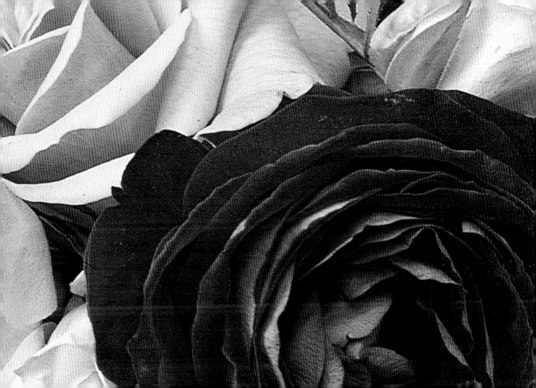

geranium

Pelargonium graveclens and *Pelargonium odorantissium*

Mind–body influence: *Balancing (stimulates or relaxes according to need)*

Sometimes known as rose geranium, geranium essential oil is extracted from the flowers and leaves of a shrub native to Madagascar. It has a sweet, floral scent and is an attractive pale green color. It is a mildly antiseptic oil that is useful for treating many skin conditions, either by adding a few drops to the bath, as a steam facial, or as a massage. Geranium is an exceptionally good oil for women and has proved helpful in alleviating period pains and

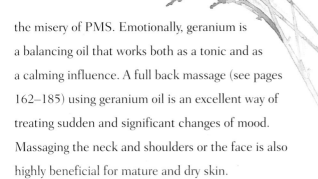

FOR A RELAXING
MASSAGE

2 drops geranium oil
2 drops rose oil
2 drops lavender oil
blended with
2 tablespoons carrier oil

the misery of PMS. Emotionally, geranium is a balancing oil that works both as a tonic and as a calming influence. A full back massage (see pages 162–185) using geranium oil is an excellent way of treating sudden and significant changes of mood. Massaging the neck and shoulders or the face is also highly beneficial for mature and dry skin.

Blending: Mixes well with most other essential oils.

Use for a face and scalp massage or for an upper back and shoulder massage. This massage will relieve anxiety and relax an overtaxed mind.

oils for women's health

Menopause A good general treatment for recapturing a level of wellbeing and reducing stress is to use 6 drops of one of the following oils—clary sage, cypress, and geranuim—in a warm bath. To help night sweats, use 1 drop of one of the oils as an inhalation on a cotton handkerchief.

PMS Soaking in a warm bath containing 1 drop of each of the following essential oils—lavender, clary sage, and geranium—before sleeping will help to ease the troublesome symptoms of PMS.

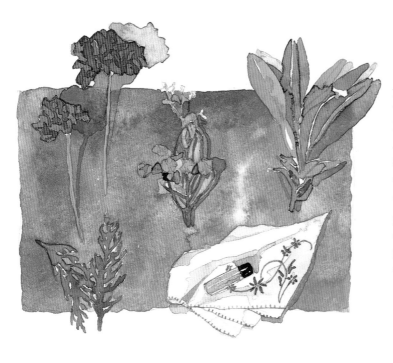

RECIPE FOR
TREATING
MENSTRUAL CRAMPS
3 drops juniper oil and
2 drops of clary sage oil
in 2–3 cups hot water

Wring out a cloth and
place over the affected
area. Renew the hot
poultice as soon as it has
cooled to blood heat.

jasmine *Jasminum officinale*

Mind–body influence: *Stimulating; Aphrodisiac*

Sometimes called the king of oils, jasmine is extracted from the flowers of the plant. Since these have to be hand-picked and it takes about 8,000 blooms to make a single gram of oil, it is understandably very expensive.

Used in a warm bath or for a gentle massage, jasmine oil is very therapeutic for all kinds of cramps, and diluted to half its usual strength, it can be helpful during labor. Its uplifting and relaxing aroma is effective in treating PMS.

Many negative feelings
can be overcome by massage, baths,
or inhalation using jasmine oil. It makes
a wonderful fragrance for a candlelit winter
interior when sprinkled on wood for a fire, and is
said to have aphrodisiac properties.

Blending: Mixes well with cedarwood,
geranium, lemon, patchouli, rose, and sandalwood.

FOR A STEAM FACIAL
*3 drops jasmine oil and
2 drops ylang ylang oil
in a bowl of hot water*

This is a good pre-
bedtime beauty
treatment, since it will
relax the mind while
rejuvenating the skin.

Lavender: Shakespeare called this fragrant flowering herb "hot lavender" because of its warming scent. Culpeper, a famous 17th-century English herbalist, described its oil as being "of a fierce and piercing quality, a very few drops being sufficient for inward or outward maladies."

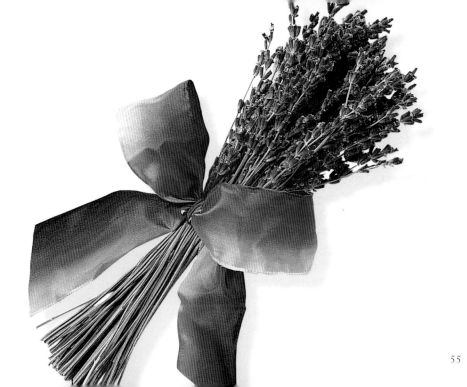

lavender

Lavendula augustifolia and *Lavendula officinalis*

Mind–body influence: *Antidepressant*

This oil comes from the flowers, leaves, and stems, and is cultivated worldwide. It is probably the best known of all the essential oils.

Lavender oil is a good antiseptic and excellent for treating infections, insect bites, and burns. Headaches—even migraine—respond well to lavender oil and inhaling a few drops on a tissue is an effective remedy for nausea. Used in a hot bath, it helps alleviate the effects of stress and

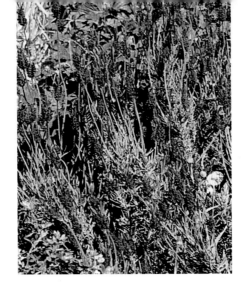

insomnia. In a lukewarm bath, it is refreshing and enlivening. Massaging with lavender oil promotes relaxation.

Blending: Mixes well with cedarwood, eucalyptus, geranium, jasmine, violet, and ylang ylang oils.

FOR A SOOTHING FOOT MASSAGE
4 drops lavender oil and 3 drops rosemary oil in 1 1/2 tablespoons carrier oil

Relaxes tired and aching feet and refreshes fatigued spirits at the same time.

neroli

Citrus bigaradia Mind–body influence: *Relaxing; Antidepressant*

Derived from the blossoms of the bitter orange tree and named after the Princess of Neroli, this essential oil has a fragrance that is both bitter and flowery. A natural tranquilizer, neroli oil is excellent for treating both long-term tension and short-term stress. It is very relaxing in any massage, and is also beneficial to the skin. The sensuous smell of neroli makes it a perfect oil for room fragrancing.

Blending: Mixes well with cedarwood, frankincense, lemon, patchouli, rose, sandalwood, and ylang ylang oils.

FOR A TRANQUILIZING BATH

2 drops neroli oil, 2 drops rose oil, 2 drops lavender oil, and 2 drops ylang ylang oil

This combination of flowery fragrances is ideal for a calming bath just before bedtime.

FOR A STEAM FACIAL FOR MATURE SKIN

2 drops neroli oil and 3 drops rose oil in a bowl of hot water

While your skin benefits from these purifying oils, let your mind gently unwind.

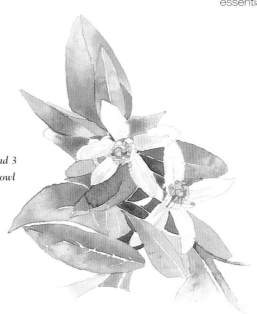

rose *Rosa centifolia* and *Rosa damascena*

Mind–body influence: *Relaxing; Antidepressant; Aphrodisiac*

Extracted from rose petals, rose oil is one of the most expensive. It has a strong yet delicate, sweet smell. Excellent for treating all kinds of depression, it is also effective against headaches and insomnia. It is also good for the skin, particularly mature skin.

A neck and face massage with rose oil is both a great beauty treatment and a wonderful lift to the spirits. A full body massage is deliciously relaxing and gives sometimes neglected areas of skin a special treat. A few drops of rose oil in a warm bath helps treat headaches, allergies, and hangovers. Rose oil also works well in an essential oil burner.

Blending: Mixes well with geranium, jasmine, lemon, neroli, patchouli, sandalwood, and ylang ylang oils.

FOR A FACE MASSAGE
*2 drops rose oil,
1 drop violet oil, and 1 drop
geranium oil in 1½
tablespoons carrier oil*

This is an excellent recipe for treating wrinkled or puffy skin. Use your fingertips only.

61

oils for mild depression

Aromatherapy can relieve the feelings of mild depression and sadness through massage. Recommended oils are basil, clary sage, Roman chamomile, rose, or thyme. You can also use these oils in a bath—choose one of the oils and add 6–8 drops to the bathwater. You can also inhale the oils through an impregnated tissue or handkerchief (3 drops on a tissue, then inhale through the nose for about 1 minute. Repeat 3 times a day.)

Try this combination of oils as an inhalation to relieve depression and anxiety. Add 3 drops of frankincense oil and 2 drops of chamomile to a bowl of hot water. Breathe deeply to leave you feeling soothed.

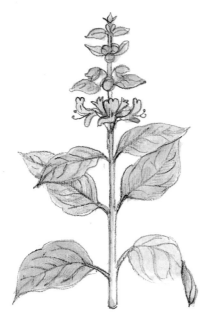

Both basil and thyme essential oils can help to uplift the spirits. Only use thyme oil in a bath, as directed opposite.

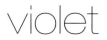 violet

Viola odorata Mind–Body influence: *Relaxing*

The oil is derived from the flowers and leaves.

It has a delicate, floral smell, and a few drops in a warm bath will clear the head and aid concentration.

A facial massage with undiluted violet oil is both pleasurable and beneficial. It is good for treating open pores, blackheads, spots, thread veins, rashes, and sore or irritated skin. It may be used for a gentle steam facial, too. Steam inhalation is also good for relieving headaches.

Blending: Mixes well with geranium, rose, and lime oils.

FOR A RELAXING BATH

4 drops violet oil, 2 drops rose oil, and 2 drops ylang ylang oil

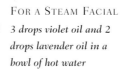

This is a good combination for easing tension and worries, and for restoring concentration.

FOR A STEAM FACIAL

3 drops violet oil and 2 drops lavender oil in a bowl of hot water

This is a deep cleansing facial that is gentle on even the driest and most delicate skin.

FOR A FACE AND NECK MASSAGE

3 drops violet oil and 2 drops rose oil in 1½ tablespoons carrier oil

Squeeze the contents of a vitamin E capsule into the mixture for extra richness.

ylang ylang *Cananga odorata*

Mind–Body influence: *Relaxing; Antidepressant; Aphrodisiac*

The oil is extracted from the flowers of a tropical tree. The name means "flower of flowers." The essential oil has a strong, sweet, floral aroma that is very sensuous. It is hypnotic and relaxing, and is therefore used for relieving all kinds of emotional turmoil. It is also sometimes a useful skin and hair treatment.

Used in an essential oil burner, ylang ylang oil creates a sensuous, romantic mood ideal for the bedroom.

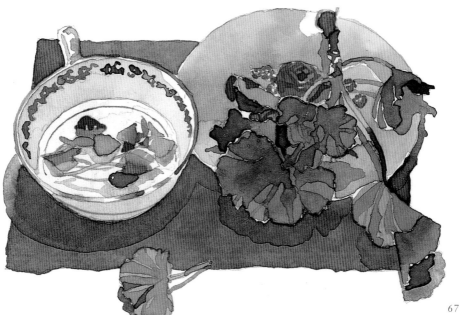

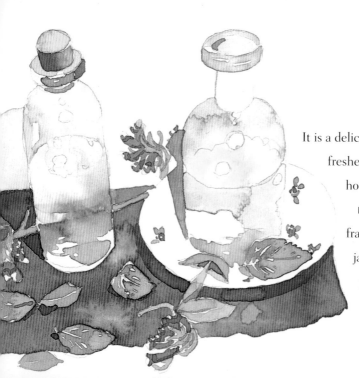

It is a deliciously aromatic room freshener in other parts of the house, too.

Blending: Mixes well with frankincense, geranium, jasmine, lemon, neroli, patchouli, petitgrain, rose, and sandalwood oils.

For a Calming Massage

4 drops ylang ylang oil, 3 drops jasmine oil, and 2 drops geranium oil in 1 1/2 tablespoons carrier oil

Use for a sensuous full body rub or hypnotically soothing back massage.

For a Relaxing Bath

4 drops ylang ylang oil and 4 drops petitgrain oil

This relieves tension after a hard day in the most luxurious way. It is especially appealing to the female nose.

For a Body Moisturizer

2 drops ylang ylang oil, 2 drops jasmine oil, and 2 drops sandalwood oil in 1 1/2 tablespoons carrier oil

This is particularly effective for dry skin on elbows and knees.

To lift yourself out of the daily grind of
existence to a state of sublime sensuousness,
add 3 drops of jasmine oil, 3 drops of sandalwood
oil, and 3 drops of ylang ylang oil to your
bathwater. Lay back and luxuriate in its intimate,
feminine fragrance. This is also an ideal
mixture for relieving stress.

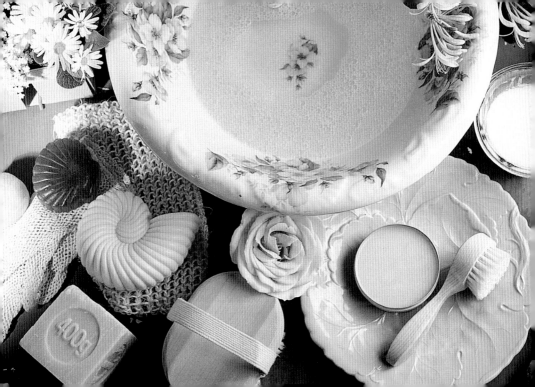

spicy oils

These oils offer a range
of interesting and complex scents,
from the warm, rich, and
inviting to the refreshing
and piquant.

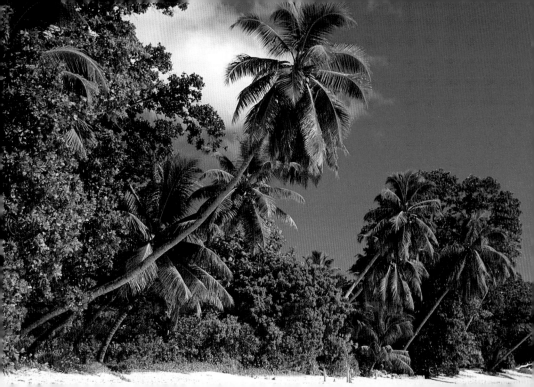

ginger *Zingiber officinalis*

Mind–body influence: *Stimulating; Aphrodisiac*

The oil is extracted from the root of a plant that grows in the Caribbean, Africa, India, and Japan, and has a warm, spicy smell. It is warming, stimulating, and also antiseptic.

It is an ideal oil for use in massage or in a bath in cold weather since it boosts the circulation. A foot massage is an excellent way of restoring tired feet.

Blending: Mixes well with bay, eucalyptus, jasmine, neroli, patchouli, and rose oils.

For Treating a Muscular Pain

3 drops ginger oil and 3 drops eucalyptus oil in 2–3 cups hot water

Squeeze out a cloth and apply the hot poultice to the affected area. It is also effective for easing a sore throat.

For a Therapeutic Bath

2 drops ginger oil, 3 drops eucalyptus oil, and 4 drops rosemary oil

Hot water and warming oils combine to ease muscular aches and pains.

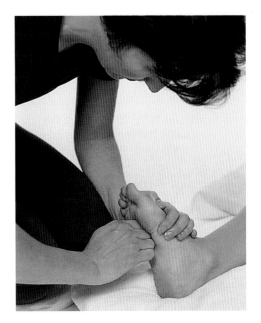

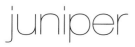 juniper

Juniperus communis Mind–body influence: *Relaxing*

The oil is extracted from the berries of the juniper tree. Juniper oil is especially effective in treating women's health problems. However, it should never be used during pregnancy. A few drops in a hot bath can help relieve the distress of PMS and menstrual cramps.

Make sure you buy essential oil of juniper, since there is a cheaper, less effective juniper oil available made from the needles and twigs of the tree rather than extracts from the berries. Massage with juniper oil is excellent for muscular

pains and rheumatism, while a brisk rub
is helpful for treating cellulite.
It is also effective for
toning oily skin.

Blending: Mixes well
with cedarwood,
eucalyptus,
frankincense, geranium,
neroli, and petitgrain oils.

FOR A
STIMULATING BATH
3 drops juniper oil and
3 drops patchouli oil

This is especially toning
in a cool or tepid bath
after the wear and tear
of a hot day.

77

myrrh

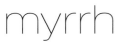

Commiphora myrrha Mind–body influence: *Relaxing*

The oil is derived from the resin of a tree native to the Middle East. The essential oil has a rich and spicy smell, and is exceptionally good for treating skin problems. It is also helpful in relieving stress.

A few drops of myrrh oil in a warm bath provide a wonderful morale boost. It is a good expectorant, so a steam inhalation is an effective way of treating a chesty cough.

Blending: Mixes well with frankincense, neroli, patchouli, rose, and sandalwood oils.

FOR A RICH MOISTURIZER

3 drops myrrh oil and 2 drops rose oil in 1 1/2 tablespoons carrier oil

This makes a good moisturizer for dry skin. Mix with peanut or almond oil for added protection.

FOR MASSAGING MATURE SKIN

2 drops myrrh oil, 2 drops lavender oil, and 2 drops neroli oil in 1 1/2 tablespoons carrier oil

Wheatgerm oil is the ideal carrier oil. Use only your fingertips to stroke the skin around the eyes and mouth.

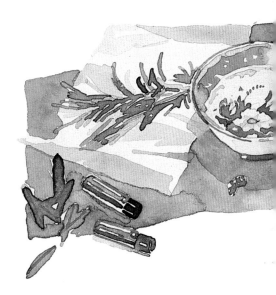

79

tea tree

Melaleuca alternifolia Mind–body influence: *Stimulating*

The oil is extracted from the leaves of an Australian shrub. It has a medicinal smell and is a non-irritating antiseptic. Tea tree is particularly effective in the treatment of fungal and viral infections, and may also be used for burns and insect stings. Tea tree is recommended for applying with a cold compress or adding to baths—it is an excellent immune-stimulant.

Blending: Mixes well with eucalyptus, geranium, lemon, and sandalwood oils.

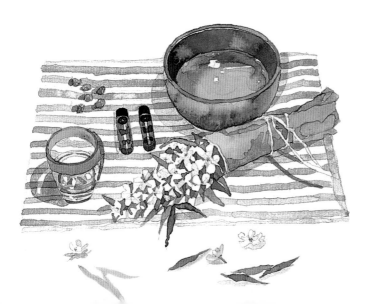

BATH FOR TREATING
COUGHS AND COLDS
*3 drops tea tree oil, 2
drops lemon oil, and 2
drops pine oil*

Relax in the hot
water, breathing in
the scented steam to
ease tightness and
congestion before
going to bed.

81

wood & herb oils

*The oils from trees
have an invigorating pine-
like or resinous scent,
while the herbaceous oils
offer a variety of aromas.*

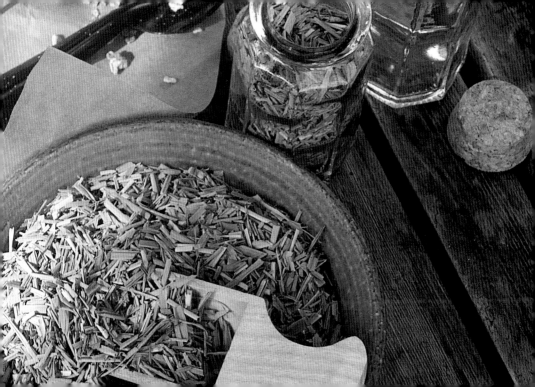

bay

Pimenta racemosa Mind–body influence: *Stimulating*

West Indian bay oil is extracted from the leaves and berries of a South American tree. The oil has a strong, woody scent. It is mildly antiseptic and strongly astringent.

This is a particularly potent oil that may irritate the nose and throat in some cases, so it should be used in moderation and very well diluted. It is good as a decongestant when inhaled with steam.

Blending: Mixes well with cedarwood, eucalyptus, lemon, and sandalwood oils.

FOR A CELLULITE RUB

2 drops bay oil, 2 drops lemon oil, and 4 drops lavender oil in 1½ tablespoons sesame oil

Massage in long, firm strokes using your palms up the thighs from the knees.

FOR A STIMULATING MASCULINE BATH

2 drops bay oil, 2 drops cedarwood oil, and 2 drops lemon oil

Use in the bath or mix with a carrier oil and apply to the skin before showering.

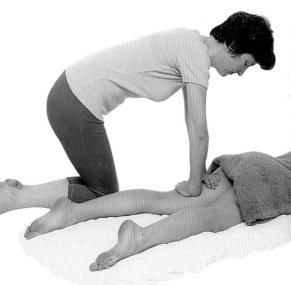

cedarwood *Juniperus virginiana*

Mind–body influence: *Relaxing*

The oil is extracted from the wood of the tree. It has a pleasant, refreshing, woody smell and is a popular fragrance with men. Its astringent properties make it an effective oil for skin conditions. It is an excellent decongestant—especially useful in treating sinus infections—and acts as a stimulating tonic used in a bath or for massage.

Blending: Mixes well with eucalyptus, frankincense, geranium, jasmine, and lemon oils.

FOR MOISTURIZING OILY SKIN

2 drops cedarwood oil and 1 drop juniper oil in 1 1/2 tablespoons carrier oil

Squeeze in the contents of a vitamin E capsule and mix well to make a light moisturizer.

FOR A SENSUOUS BATH

3 drops cedarwood oil, 2 drops frankincense oil, and 2 drops lime oil

This is a deliciously stimulating combination of woody, spicy, and citrus smells to tone up both body and mind.

A COMPRESS FOR SKIN RASH

3 drops cedarwood oil and 2 drops lavender oil in 2–3 cups iced water

Wring out a cloth and place over the affected area. Renew when the cloth warms to blood heat.

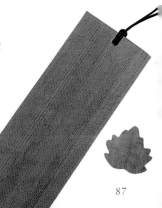

87

chamomile *Matricaria recutita* or *M. chamomilla*

and *Anthemis nobilis* Mind–body influence: *Relaxing*

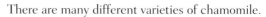

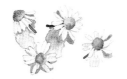

There are many different varieties of chamomile.
Chamomile is one of the gentlest and most soothing of all
the essential oils. It is naturally anti-inflammatory and can
safely be used to treat skin rashes and other problems. Its
sedative effects can benefit those suffering from headaches
and menstrual or menopausal problems.

Blending: Mixes well with cedarwood, eucalyptus,
frankincense, geranium, jasmine, and sandalwood oils.

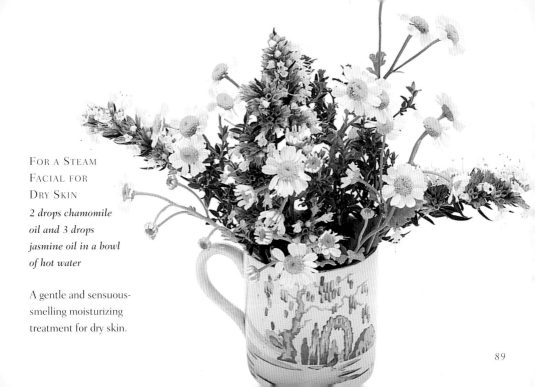

FOR A STEAM
FACIAL FOR
DRY SKIN

*2 drops chamomile
oil and 3 drops
jasmine oil in a bowl
of hot water*

A gentle and sensuous-
smelling moisturizing
treatment for dry skin.

89

*C*ome into the garden Maud,

I am here at the gate alone;

And the woodbine spices are wafted

abroad and the musk of the rose is blown.

ALFRED LORD TENNYSON: *Maud* (1855)

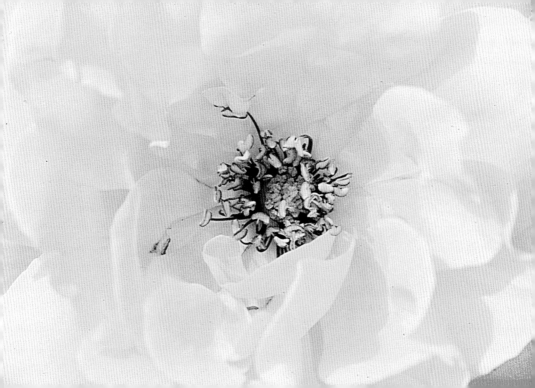

clary sage *Salvia sclarea*

Mind–body influence: *Relaxing; Antidepressant*

Although clary sage is a member of the sage family, it should not be confused with sage (*Salvia officinalis*), which produces an essential oil not recommended for home use. The oil is derived from the tips of the leaves and has an attractive nutty smell. It is excellent for treating exhaustion and may be applied as a massage oil or in a bath. Its scent has a euphoric effect, so it is good for tackling phobias, depression, and listlessness. A massage with the oil can be

helpful for both counteracting feelings of negativity
and arousing the emotions.

A warm bath with a few drops of the oil can relieve
PMS and is also effective for other aches and pains. A
face and scalp massage is helpful for tension headaches.
It is also good for skin conditions.

Blending: Mixes well with patchouli, rose, sandalwood,
and ylang ylang oils.

FOR A COMPRESS
TO REDUCE
INFLAMMATION
*3 drops clary sage and 2
drops geranium oil in
2–3 cups iced water*

As the soothing oils go
to work on the body,
their scents relax and
uplift the mind.

oils for anxiety & distress

Several essential oils will help to relieve many of the symptoms associated with anxiety, and the following oils may be used either for massage, with 4 drops in 1½ tablespoons carrier oil, or as an inhalant using 3 drops on a handkerchief inhaled through the nose for 1 minute.

For panic attacks: Clary sage, lavender, or sandalwood oils.

For tension headaches: Marjoram or chamomile oil.

As an aid to relaxation: Frankincense and patchouli oils.

An aromatic full body or back massage with ylang ylang oil can calm tension and counteract negativity, while a few drops of the oil in the bath can alleviate fears and reduce stress.

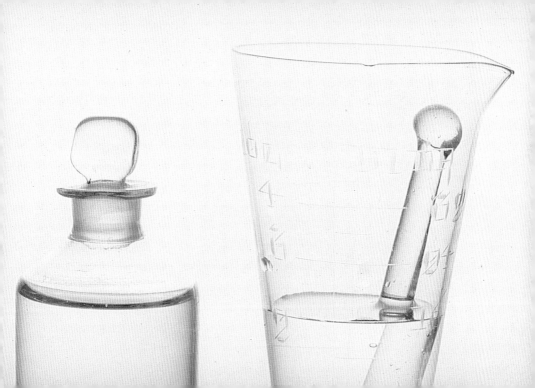

cypress

Cupressus semperverens Mind–body influence: *Relaxing*

The oil is distilled from the leaves and cones of this
Mediterranean tree.

Cypress oil is most helpful with menstrual and
menopausal problems, and can be used to treat both fluid
retention and cellulite. It is a vasoconstrictor and can be
helpful in treating varicose and broken veins.

Cypress oil is excellent for massaging the abdominal area
and relieving discomfort. A bath with a few drops of cypress
oil relieves the discomfort of piles. Menstrual problems are

best dealt with by means of a hot poultice or an aromatic bath.

The smell of cypress oil is generally regarded as too overpowering to use as a room freshener, but a few drops of the oil on a pillow at night will ease breathing and stop coughing, and can be helpful in preventing bedwetting.

Blending: Mixes well with bay, cedarwood, frankincense, geranium, lemon, and sandalwood oils.

FOR A PAIN-RELIEVING BATH
3 drops cypress oil, 2 drops geranium oil, and 2 drops lavender oil

This combination can relieve the discomfort of menstrual problems or chestiness.

eucalyptus *Eucalyptus globulus*

Mind–body influence: *Stimulating*

The oil is extracted from the twigs and leaves of the Australian gum tree. Eucalyptus has a distinctive aroma that instantly clears the head. Its decongestant effect has been employed in countless cold and cough remedies. It is a powerful antiseptic and is a warming oil for soothing muscular pains. Steam inhalation of a few drops of the oil on the pillow at night can relieve cold and flu symptoms, and help bronchitis. Heating eucalyptus oil in a vaporizer at night will help to make breathing easier and disinfect the air. It can also be applied as a chest rub, provided it is properly diluted with a carrier oil, or as a hot poultice. Eucalyptus helps heal sprains if it is properly diluted with a carrier oil and massaged directly onto the affected area.

Blending: Best used by itself, but can be mixed with bay, cedarwood, geranium, lemon, and sandalwood oils.

oils for aching muscles

To help relieve aching muscles after over-exercising, either massage essential oils, properly diluted with a carrier oil, directly into the problem areas or use in a bath. Recommended oils are chamomile, cypress, eucalyptus, and rosemary.

Add 10 drops of one of these to a bath, or 3 drops of one of the oils to 1½ tablespoons of almond oil for massage.

For massaging aching feet, blend 2 drops of chamomile oil and 2 drops of eucalyptus oil with 1½ tablespoons of carrier oil. Use this combination to soothe and revive your abused feet—see pages 188–201 for step-by-step instructions for a complete foot massage.

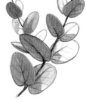

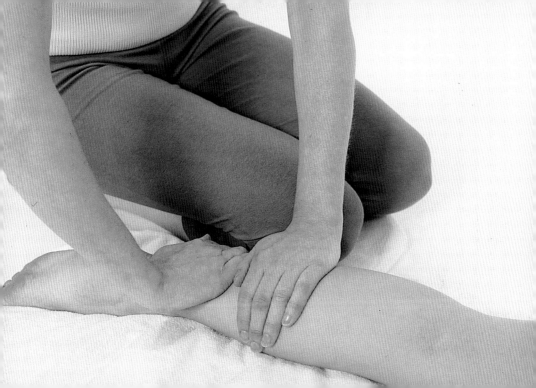

frankincense

Boswellia carteri or *Boswellia thurifera*

Mind–body influence: *Balancing (stimulates or relaxes according to need)*

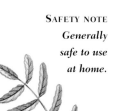

SAFETY NOTE
Generally safe to use at home.

The oil is extracted from the gum of a North African tree. Frankincense oil is especially useful in dealing with many of the symptoms of distress and panic. It helps restore a normal breathing rate and calms general nervousness. It is an excellent oil to use if you are feeling irritable, and is warming and comforting.

A face, neck, and scalp massage with the oil provides effective relief from tension headaches, while steam

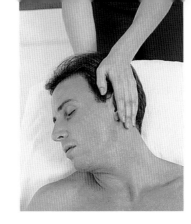

inhalation is helpful for restoring good humor. A warm bath with a few drops of frankincense oil counteracts the effects of nightmares and sudden fears. It is often described as a rejuvenating oil.

Blending: Mixes well with cedarwood, eucalyptus, geranium, lime, neroli, and patchouli oils.

FOR TREATING STRETCH MARKS
*1 drop frankincense oil,
1 drop sandalwood oil,
and 2 drops lavender oil*

Apply to the affected area and rub in gently with the fingertips.

galbanum *Feurla galbaniflua*

Mind–body influence: *Relaxing; Aphrodisiac*

The oil is derived from a resinous gum. It is cultivated in the Mediterranean and North Africa.

The essential oil has a warm, woody smell. It is relaxing and soothing, and makes a good stress-reliever. It has a tonic effect and is useful in combating fatigue. Grazed and blemished skin responds well to it.

Mixed with other oils, such as frankincense or violet, it is excellent for a therapeutic face and neck massage. Mixed with chamomile or neroli, it is good for a shoulder or back massage to relieve nervous tension. It may also be added to a warm bath, mixed with other oils, such as lavender. Inhaling a few drops on a handkerchief is an effective tonic.

Blending: Mixes well with frankincense, geranium, neroli, rose, and violet oils.

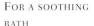

FOR A SOOTHING
BATH
2 drops galbanum oil, 2 drops geranium oil, and 2 drops lavender oil

This combination of relaxing, calming, and balancing oils is excellent for relieving frustration or anxiety.

patchouli *Pogostemon patchouli* or *Pogostemon cablin*

Mind–body influence: *Relaxing; Antidepressant; Aphrodisiac*

The oil is extracted from the leaves and shoots of an Indian herb similar to lavender. The fragrance is sweet, earthy, and very persistent.

Patchouli oil is antiseptic and anti-inflammatory, so it is good for treating cracked skin, burns, and scalp problems. Steam facials, hot poultices, cold compresses, and aromatic baths are all effective.

Used in very small quantities, patchouli oil tends to be

stimulating. In larger amounts, relatively speaking, it is relaxing. The oil is particularly useful, therefore, for treating tension and apprehension.

Blending: Mixes well with frankincense, rose, sandalwood, and ylang ylang oils.

FOR A MOISTURIZER IN WINTER WEATHER
2 drops patchouli oil, 2 drops sandalwood oil, and 2 drops myrrh oil in 1 1/2 tablespoons carrier oil

Protect your skin against the elements with this moisturizer. Use almond for sensitive skin and sunflower oil if you have an oily skin.

Patchouli oil has a heady, pungent fragrance that many people find intoxicating. For a truly sensual and sublime body massage, combine 2 drops of patchouli oil with 3 drops of geranium oil and 3 drops of rose oil, and blend with 1½ tablespoons of almond carrier oil. Now draw the curtains, light some suitably seductive scented candles, apply, and enjoy!

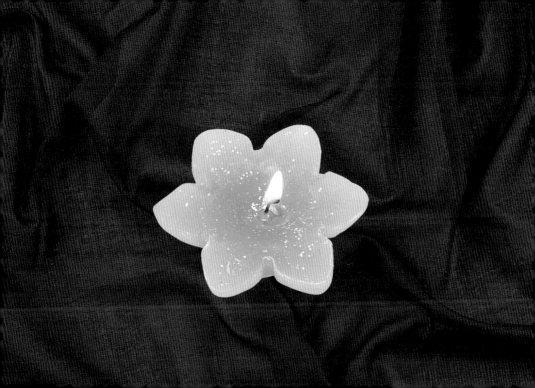

peppermint *Mentha piperata*

Mind–body influence: *Stimulating*

The oil is derived from the leaves and flowers of the herb. The essential oil is refreshing and cooling, so it is excellent for treating all kinds of pains, sore skin, insect bites, and menopausal hot flushes. Its strong menthol smell is stimulating and it is helpful for overcoming fatigue, headaches, PMS, and nausea.

Irritated skin can be soothed by soaking in a bath with peppermint oil. Use only 1 or 2 drops, since the oil is very potent. A cold compress can also be applied to the affected area. Peppermint oil is a natural and effective painkiller, so baths, hot poultices, and cold compresses are also helpful in treating various aches and pains. It is an ideal oil for a footbath or foot massage.

Blending: Mixes well with cedarwood, eucalyptus, geranium, lemon, patchouli, rose, and sandalwood oils.

FOR A STIMULATING BODY RUB

1 drop peppermint oil, 1 drop myrrh oil, and 2 drops lavender oil in 1 1/2 tablespoons carrier oil

A warming massage that you can do yourself and is an excellent start to a winter's day.

pine

Pinus sylvestris Mind–body influence: *Stimulating*

SAFETY NOTE
Generally safe for home use.

The oil is extracted from the needles of several different species of pine tree. The stimulating, balsamic aroma has a long tradition of use against respiratory infections and pine oil remains one of the best inhalants. Massage the chest with diluted pine oil for treating bronchitis, colds, and a blocked-up nose. Or add a few drops of the oil to a warm bath and allow the aromatic steam plenty of time to work. This also helps relieve the pain of arthritis, rheumatism, and muscular tension, as does gentle massage. Pine is a good oil for a hot poultice. It may be applied to the chest or to swollen joints and aching muscles. It is useful around the home because of its deodorizing and antiseptic properties.

Blending: Mixes well with cedarwood, eucalyptus, frankincense, lemon, and patchouli oils.

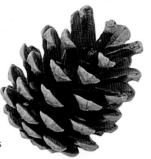

FOR A PAIN-RELIEVING MASSAGE
3 drops pine oil, 3 drops eucalyptus oil, and 3 drops frankincense oil in 1 1/2 tablespoons carrier oil

Rub gently into sore joints, but you can use firmer strokes for easing aching muscles.

rosemary

Rosemarinus officinalis

Mind–body influence: *Stimulating*

The oil is extracted from the flower tops and leaves of the herb. It has a fresh, woody scent that is stimulating for both body and mind. A bath with a few drops of rosemary oil is an excellent tonic for lethargy and poor concentration. Its strong, minty aroma is helpful in alleviating the symptoms of bronchitis and other breathing problems.

Rosemary oil has very warming properties, and a massage with it is a good way to treat muscular aches. Other "cold" conditions that respond well to rosemary are chilblains and poor circulation. Many shampoos incorporate rosemary oil in their ingredients. For home hair care, add 2 or 3 drops to the final rinse for glossy, healthy hair.

Blending: Mixes well with bay, eucalyptus, lemon, lime, neroli, and sandalwood oils.

FOR A HOME HAIR TREATMENT
2 drops rosemary oil, 1 drop lavender oil, and 1 drop bay oil in 1 1/2 tablespoons almond or olive oil

Use for a scalp massage, working the mixture well into the roots of your hair. Cover and leave for 30 minutes before shampooing as normal.

To create a wonderfully warming, inviting,
and festive atmosphere at Christmas,
make a fragrant wood fire. Use 4 drops of
ginger oil, 4 drops of sandalwood oil, and
4 drops of orange oil sprinkled

on 3 or 4 logs of wood. Let them absorb the oils for about 15 minutes before lighting the fire. The spicy aroma will immediately get your family and other guests in the party mood.

sandalwood *Santalum album*

Mind–body influence: *Relaxing; Antidepressant; Aphrodisiac*

SAFETY NOTE
Generally safe for home use.

The oil is derived from the roots and wood of the tree. It has a sweet, woody smell that has been used in perfumes for many centuries.

This is a deliciously sensuous oil, and a full body massage is a treat. It helps relieve listlessness, insecurity, and tension, and also helps restore a loss of libido. An added bonus is that the oil is good for dry or chapped skin. A warm bath with a few drops of sandalwood oil is deeply relaxing and helps insomnia.

The oil is good for treating coughs, colds, and congestion. A hot bath or steam inhalation helps clear mucus, and a hot poultice relieves the pain of a sore throat. It is an excellent choice as a room freshener and is one of the best oils for scenting a wood fire.

Blending: Mixes well with frankincense, geranium, jasmine, patchouli, petitgrain, and rose oils.

FOR A BEDTIME MASSAGE
3 drops sandalwood oil and 2 drops chamomile oil in 1 1/2 tablespoons carrier oil

A soothing massage of shoulders, scalp, forehead, and temples should provide a night of sweet dreams.

stress-relief

The following essential oils are beneficial for relieving the effects of stress and exhaustion: vetiver, chamomile, lavender, and neroli. The most relaxing of all baths is the "neutral" bath, where the water is more or less equal to body temperature and the bath is best taken just before bedtime.

Allow a period of 20 minutes for your aromatic neutral bath. For maximum benefit, as much of the body should be submerged as possible. Periodic topping-up with hot water is usually necessary to prevent the water from cooling. It is also important to make sure the bathroom is warm so that stepping out is not a shock.

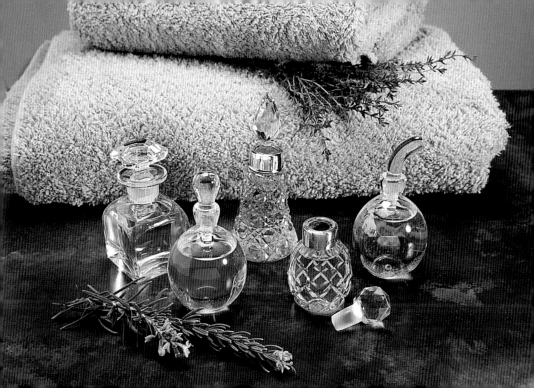

6 citrus oils

*These oils capture all
the tangy freshness and
revitalizing zestfulness of the
fruits they come from.*

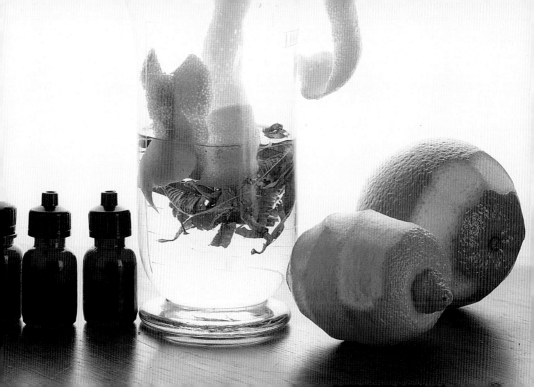

bergamot

Citrus bergamia Mind–body influence: *Balancing (stimulates or relaxes according to need); Antidepressant*

The oil is extracted from the rind of a small orange-like fruit from Italy. It has a light, uplifting scent and is good for treating anxiety and negativity. It is mildly antiseptic and very helpful with most aspects of skin care. It is an effective deodorizer, which makes it an excellent choice for scenting a room. It is good for ridding clothes of persistent body odors; simply sprinkle a few drops along the seams. At times of stress, discreetly sniffing a few drops on a handkerchief will do wonders for your confidence. This is also effective against travel sickness.

Blending: Mixes well with bay, lemon, lime, neroli, sandalwood, and ylang ylang oils.

FOR AN INVIGORATING BATH

3 drops bergamot oil, 3 drops petitgrain oil, and 2 drops lemon oil

Stirred into a warm bath, this recipe is guaranteed to banish the winter blues.

lemon 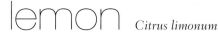 *Citrus limonum*

Mind–body influence: *Stimulating; Antidepressant*

The oil is extracted from the rind of the fruit. It has a tangy, citrus scent that is refreshing and invigorating, and is a good pick-me-up first thing in the morning or whenever you are feeling under the weather. It is antiseptic and strongly astringent, and has a reputation for treating warts and corns. A hot poultice prepared with a few drops of lemon oil performs wonders for tired and aching feet.

The fresh-smelling oil is excellent for banishing the "cobwebs," and inhaling a few drops on a handkerchief

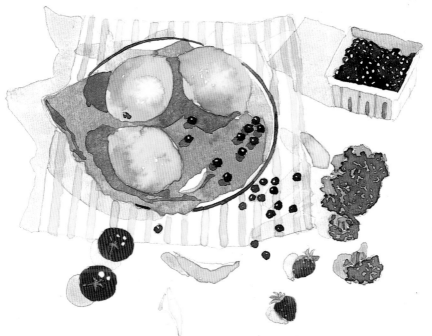

clears the head. A hot citrusy bath on a cold winter night stimulates the circulation. Massage with lemon oil will leave you feeling energized and is also a good treatment for cellulite. Its fresh, clean smell makes lemon oil ideal for use around the house.

Blending: Lemon oil does not mix well with many other essential oils because of its highly distinctive, overpowering fragrance.

FOR MASSAGING
FEET WITH CORNS OR
PLANTER WARTS
*2 drops lemon oil and 3
drops tea tree oil in 1 1/2
tablespoons carrier oil*

This can be effective if
used over a period of
time, but will not work
magic overnight.

FOR A STIMULATING
SUMMER BATH
*3 drops lemon, 3 drops
rosemary oil, and 3
drops peppermint oil*

A cool bath is a real
pick-me-up after a hot,
tiring day.

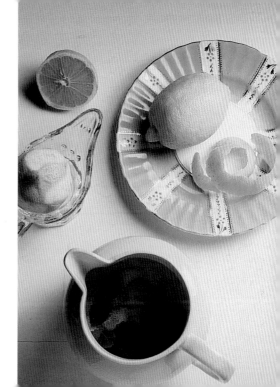

remedies
for coughs & colds

Head colds: The use of essential oils in a bath or a steam inhalation can help relieve that "blocked-up feeling" in the head and ease the pain in the sinuses.

Use 2 drops of eucalyptus, lemon, or cedarwood oil added to your bath water or to a bowl of hot water for inhalation, or add 2 drops of one of these oils to 1½ tablespoons of carrier oil (see pages 152–153) and rub on the upper chest.

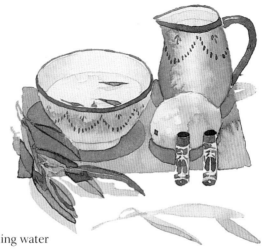

Coughs: Add 3 drops of one of the following essential oils—eucalyptus, thyme, cypress, and sandalwood—to a bowl of steaming water as an inhalation. Inhale for more than 10 minutes. Repeat up to 3 times a day **Safety note:** These cough treatments are recommended for adults only.

Use eucalyptus and lemon oils in a steam inhalation for head colds.

lemongrass *Cymbopogon citratus*

Mind–body influence: *Stimulating*

The oil is extracted from a wild grass that is now widely cultivated for the perfume industry. It has a warm, citrus smell that is less sharp than lemon oil.

It is an excellent choice for treating skin eruptions and can also heal areas of inflammation. It can be used for a stimulating aromatic shower. Mix with a carrier oil as for massage and rub into your skin before getting under the water. It is ideal for adding to baths since it will boost

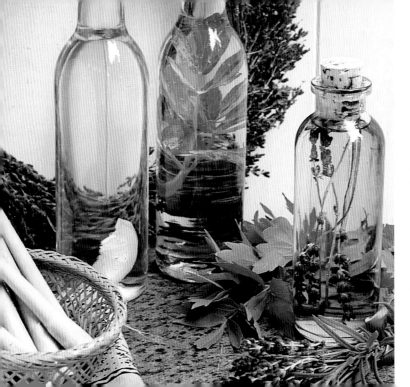

Add a few drops
of lemongrass oil
to a cotton ball
and place inside
the garbage can
to both deodorize
and keep away
flies and wasps.

133

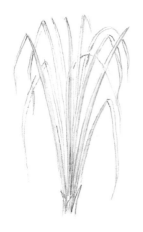

circulation and help control excessive perspiration. Its deodorizing properties also make it a useful room freshener. Lemongrass oil is an effective insect repellent. Its advantage over citronella is that it does not smell as powerfully. You can apply it diluted in a carrier oil to your skin, or alternatively, for use indoors, sprinkle a few drops on the hems of drapes.

Blending: Mixes well with frankincense, geranium, and jasmine oils.

FOR A THERAPEUTIC FOOTBATH

4 drops lemongrass oil and 4 drops lavender oil in a large bowl of hot water

Use this to control excessive perspiration of the feet—or hands.

FOR A STIMULATING MASSAGE

2 drops lemongrass oil, 3 drops orange oil, and 1 drop rosemary oil in 1 1/2 tablespoons carrier oil

This summery combination of oils is ideal for a back or shoulder massage.

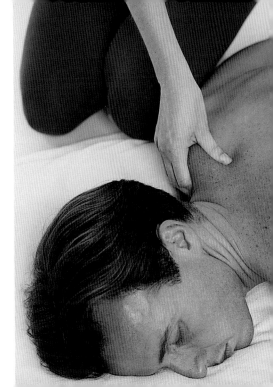

lime *Citrus aurantifolia* Mind–body influence: *Stimulating; Antidepressant*

The oil is extracted from the rind of the fruit before it ripens. It has a sweet citrus smell that is not quite as sharp as lemon oil, and is especially appealing to men. It is a warming and stimulating oil with antiseptic properties.

A vigorous massage with lime oil is excellent for treating poor circulation and cellulite. A few drops of the oil in a warm bath is also effective in helping these conditions and relieves the symptoms of colds and flu.

Properly diluted in a carrier oil, lime oil may be rubbed on the chest to relieve colds and coughs, on aching joints to relieve rheumatism, or as an astringent on greasy skin. Steam inhalation reduces breathing problems.

Blending: Mixes well with cedarwood, frankincense, geranium, lemon, and violet oils.

FOR A REVIVING FOOT MASSAGE
2 drops lime oil and 2 drops cedarwood oil in 1 1/2 tablespoons carrier oil

You can rub the soles of your feet vigorously, but use only light palm strokes and fingertips on ankles and shins.

137

The therapeutic as well as the cosmetic properties
of the orange were exploited by the Indians and Chinese
more than 4,000 years ago. During the numerous and
devastating outbreaks of bubonic plague across Europe in the
Middle Ages, oranges stuck with cloves were used to ward off
the disease. Queen Elizabeth 1 of England was reputed to
have worn one around her neck. Today, pomanders such as
these are often used as Christmas tree decorations.

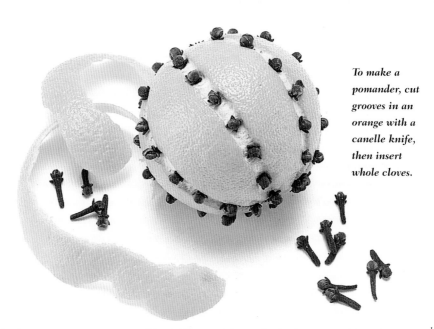

To make a pomander, cut grooves in an orange with a canelle knife, then insert whole cloves.

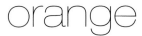 # orange *Citrus sinensis* and *Citrus aurantium*

Mind–body influence: *Antidepressant*

The oil is extracted from the rind of the fruit. Its fruity smell is cheering and refreshing. An excellent oil for reviving the spirits and dealing with lack of energy, it also has a rejuvenating effect on the skin.

An orange-oil massage is an excellent pick-me-up at the end of a working day before a busy evening. It refreshes and calms, but without sending you to sleep. A warm bath with orange oil will have a similar effect. A timesaving refresher when you are rushing from one appointment to another is to relax with a cold orange oil compress, preferably lying down with the feet raised.

It is a delicious oil for scenting a wood fire, which is a subtle way of calming fractious children. (Orange oil should not

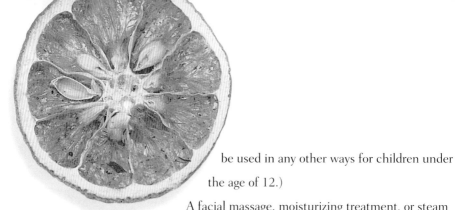

be used in any other ways for children under the age of 12.)

A facial massage, moisturizing treatment, or steam facial using orange oil will benefit a dull complexion and help smooth away wrinkles. It also makes an excellent body moisturizer, but should be used in moderation.

Orange oil only retains its therapeutic value for a maximum of 6–8 months.

Blending: Mixes well with cedarwood, lemon, myrrh, patchouli, and sandalwood oils.

FOR A REVIVING BATH

2 drops orange oil, 2 drops frankincense oil, and 2 drops geranium oil

Soak in a warm bath with this combination of oils and you will step out feeling radiant and rejuvenated.

FOR A RICH MOISTURIZER

2 drops orange oil, 1 drop lemon oil, and 1 drop lime oil in 1½ tablespoons carrier oil

This is an excellent mixture for thread veins or a dull and sallow complexion. Using

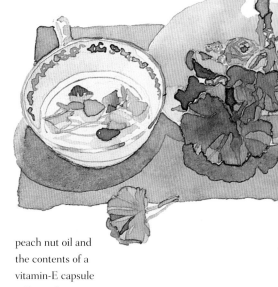

peach nut oil and the contents of a vitamin-E capsule will enrich it.

petitgrain *Citrus aurantium amara*

Mind–body influence: *Antidepressant*

The oil is derived from the leaves and twigs of the bitter orange tree. It has a sharp orange smell. Its tangy aroma is both relaxing and stimulating, so it is an excellent oil for counteracting sluggishness, fatigue, insomnia, and tension.

A shoulder and neck or back massage with petitgrain oil is an effective remedy for muscular or nervous tension. To counteract fatigue and help cure insomnia, a bath with a few drops of the oil is both relaxing and pampering. Inhale a

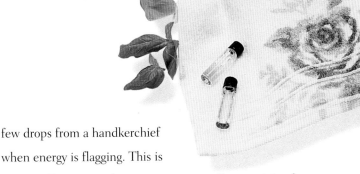

few drops from a handkerchief when energy is flagging. This is also an effective antidote to nervousness. For a reviving face mask, combine 2 drops of the oil with 2 drops of lemon and 2 drops of ylang ylang oil in 1½ tablespoons of iced water. Mix with ground almonds to make a smooth paste.

Blending: Mixes well with eucalyptus, lemon, lime, sandalwood, and ylang ylang oils.

FOR RELIEVING
MUSCULAR PAINS
*3 drops petitgrain oil
and 2 drops eucalyptus
oil in 2–3 cups hot
water*

Wring out a cloth and apply as a hot poultice to areas of muscular tension or cramps.

145

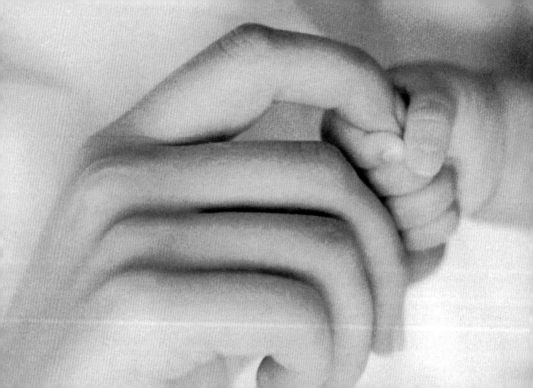

the healing
touch

the magic of massage

Touch is an instinctive human response to comfort and soothe, yet in modern society we tend to try to avoid coming into physical contact with other people. Massage is a wonderful way to harness the healing power of touch.

Massage communicates a sense of peace and develops a feeling of being in touch with our inner selves. The action of rubbing

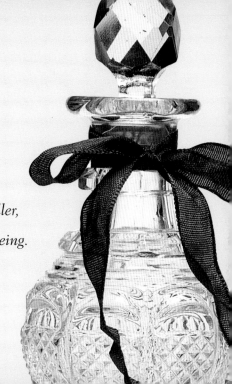

the skin creates changes in the body and the

hormone endorphin, the body's natural painkiller,

is released, which also imparts a sense of wellbeing.

Massage improves circulation and encourages

muscles to relax and extend, relieving tension

and releasing toxins from the body.

*T*he various physical, mental, and emotional responses to stress can be alleviated by healthy living and particularly the ability to relax. Through the act of relaxation, we stimulate a part of the brain that slows down both the heart rate and the rate of breathing, lowers blood pressure, and stimulates digestion and the immune system. Massage can be one of the most effective ways to learn how to relax.

GILL TREE, *Director of Essentials for Health, school of massage*

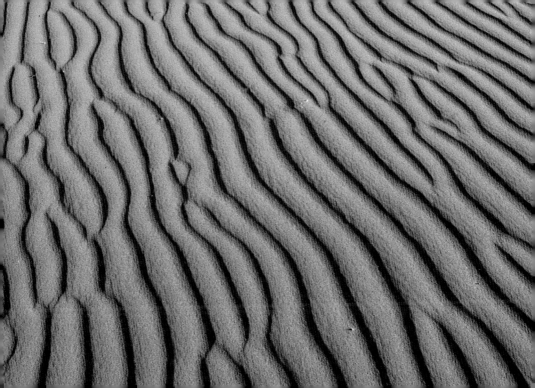

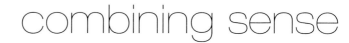

combining sense

Essential oils are beneficial in massage not only through our sense of smell but also due to the chemical properties of the oils, which enter the body through the skin. Essential oils should never be used undiluted on the skin, but always diluted in a vegetable carrier oil (see page 154).

Massage carrier oils Good-quality unrefined, cold-pressed, additive-free vegetable oils are the most suitable. Choose from sweet almond, apricot kernel, avocado, grapeseed, safflower, and

& touch

sunflower oil. Nut oils should be strictly avoided by anyone with an allergy to nuts, but all oils should be tested on the skin in case of an allergic reaction.

Always carry out a patch test on the inside of the elbow or wrist when an essential oil is being used for the first time. A rash will usually appear within 24 hours if the skin does react negatively, in which case try an alternative oil. Pour the oil into the palm of your hand to warm it before applying it to the skin.

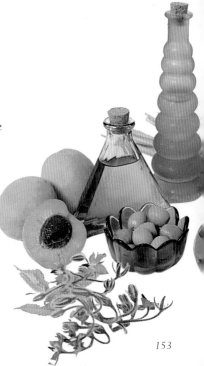

essential oils for
massage

The following essential oils are the safest and most beneficial to use for

Always dilute with a carrier vegetable oil at the ratio of 1 drop of essential oil per teaspoon of carrier oil.

Bergamot: Good for all stress-related conditions and skin problems. Safety: avoid sunlight after use, since it increases the skin's photosensitivity.

Clary sage: A relaxing yet uplifting oil. Safety: not to be used during pregnancy or if drinking alcohol; care should be taken if

stress-relieving massage.

you are driving after use.

Geranium: Has a balancing and
regulating effect on both mind and
body. Safety: generally safe, but may cause
skin sensitization in some individuals.

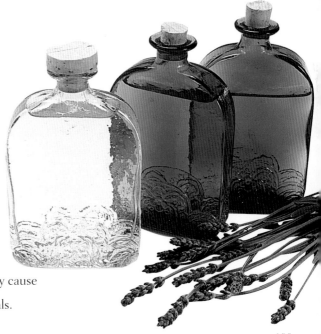

Ginger: Good for muscular and rheumatic conditions. Safety: may cause skin sensitization; avoid during pregnancy where there is high blood pressure.

Lavender: A popular oil for relieving stress, depression, and headaches. Safety: not to be used during the first three months of pregnancy.

Mandarin: Lifts the spirit and imparts a sense of peace and joy. Safety: may be phototoxic.

Neroli: Soothing to the nervous system; good for insomnia.

Peppermint: A strong-smelling oil that has a simulating effect on the nervous system. Safety: use in moderation and avoid during pregnancy or if taking homeopathic remedies; may cause skin sensitization.

Roman chamomile: Calms fragile nerves, helps promote sleep, and soothes irritated skin. Safety: may cause skin sensitization in some individuals; avoid during pregnancy.

Rosemary: Refreshing and stimulating, especially for a fatigued mind or body. Safety: not to be used in cases of pregnancy, epilepsy, and high blood pressure.

Sandalwood: Excellent for stress-related problems, skin conditions, and bronchial problems.

Sweet marjoram: Eases colds and coughs, and muscular and rheumatic aches and pains. Safety: avoid during pregnancy.

Tea tree: An excellent immune-stimulant, and helps to combat a wide range of infections. Safety: may cause skin sensitization in some individuals.

Ylang ylang: A calming and uplifting oil. Good for stress-related conditions including depression, shock, and insomnia. Safety: an excess may cause headaches and nausea; may cause skin sensitization.

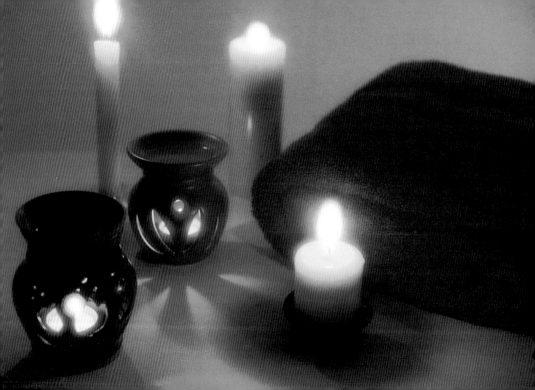

making preparations

To make your massage as effective and pleasurable as possible, first find a room that is quiet and large enough for your partner or whoever you are massaging to lie down and for you to move all around their body. The room should also be warmer than usual, since people often become chilled as they relax and their body systems slow. Cover them with warm towels and uncover only the parts of the body that you are massaging at the time.

Create a soothing atmosphere by having subdued lighting or candlelight. Perfume the air with an essential oil that complements your choice of oils for the massage. Put 5–6 drops of the oil in some water in an essential oil burner half an hour before you begin the massage.

massage safety

Always treat the person you are massaging with tender, loving care and focus on the quality of your massage rather than talking. Always check whether you are causing pain and how effective your techniques are. Never put pressure on bones or joints, and soothe with effleurage (see pages 164–169) after giving a deep massage.

After the massage, encourage your partner to get up slowly since they may feel a little light-headed. Make sure they drink plenty of water to flush out waste products released during the massage. Warn them that it is normal to ache a little after the massage.

It is always advisable to get permission from an individual's medical practitioner before giving them a massage if there is any doubt about the condition of their health. Massage is generally a very safe therapy, but there are some health conditions where it is inadvisable—see the panel on the right.

CONDITIONS INADVISABLE FOR MASSAGE

- *Varicose veins and thrombosis—never massage deeply over a varicose vein*
- *Heart conditions*
- *Inflammations, skin infections, or bruising*
- *Scar tissue*
- *Fever*
- *Recent injuries*
- *Do not massage the lower back during pregnancy*
- *Any inflamed disease or condition*
- *Cancer*
- *Arthritis*

a full back massage

Massaging the back is the most effective way to relax the whole body by stimulating the nerves emanating from the spinal cord. This area of the body suffers most from stress and neglect, including backache due to poor posture and knotted muscles from tension. Therefore, it is the best area of the body to focus on in massage to produce complete all-over relaxation.

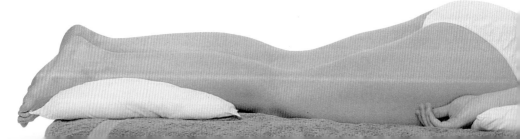

The comfort of your partner or the person receiving the massage is vital to a relaxing massage. They should be lying face down— carefully positioned pillows can make lying on the floor more comfortable. Experiment with a small pillow under the abdomen and/or chest, one under the head, and another under the calves. A rolled-up towel or bolster would be equally useful. If comfortable, the best position for the arms is by the sides.

Uncover the whole back, keeping the legs covered with towels. Position yourself at the head, and apply carrier oil blended with an essential oil (see pages 154–157) to the back in gentle, even strokes, making sure you cover the sides, neck, and under the shoulders.

effleurage

This is a soothing, rhythmic stroke used to relax the body at the beginning and end of a massage.

Effleurage accustoms your partner to you and your hands, and provides you with information about your partner—how much pressure they like, whether they are ticklish, and where they hold their tension.

Effleurage is performed by stroking toward the heart and toward the lymph nodes to assist the return of blood and lymphatic drainage. The depth of the manipulation given pushes blood toward the skin to feed it with both oxygen and nutrients.

It precedes all other strokes because of its relaxing effect, both psychologically and physiologically, and it prepares muscles for deeper manipulations. It also follows other strokes to increase blood and lymph flow into and out of the massaged area, removing waste products and toxins.

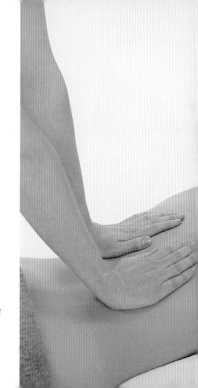

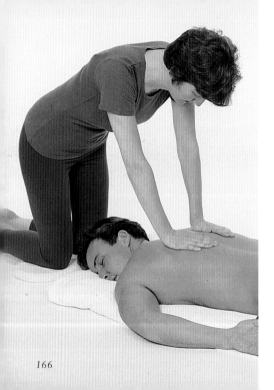

1. Place your hands on the upper back with fingers and thumbs together, pointing down the back on each side of the spine, with the thumbs about 1½ inches apart. Be careful never to apply pressure directly on the spine. Keeping your hands parallel and relaxed, glide them firmly down the back on each side of the spine at a slow and even pace, leaning in with your body weight. Make sure there is firm and equal pressure throughout your palms.

2. As you reach the lower back, turn your hands so they sweep out toward the hips, ready to glide up the sides of your partner's back.

3. As you bring your hands up the sides of the back, lean backward so you can use your body weight to assist you. Again keeping your thumbs together, try to maintain as much contact as possible. Take care not to quicken the pace as you glide your hands toward the shoulder joints. This return stroke can be applied lightly for greater relaxation or more firmly to stimulate the muscles of the sides of the back.

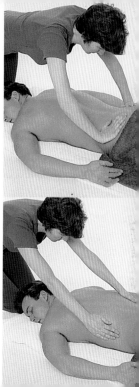

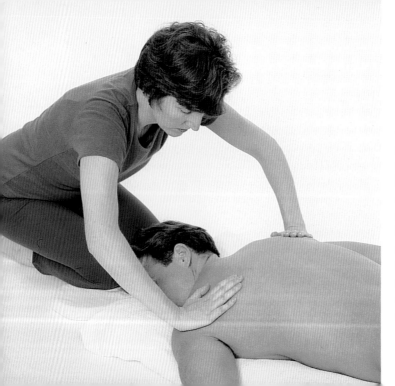

4. Lighten the pressure on reaching the shoulders and turn your hands so your wrists and elbows are pointing outward. Cupping your hands around the contours of the body, take your hands down the top of the arms to about halfway down the upper arm.

5. From there, turn your hands 180 degrees so your wrists are leading your fingers back up the arm. Let your fingers scoop underneath the shoulders and extend your fingertips so they are strong and rigid to scoop deeply into the shoulder muscles. Using only your fingers, not the thumbs, imagine your hands are blades rotating into the muscles. This is an area of great tension in most people, and your partner will appreciate deeper pressure to help release the tension and tightness.

6. Glide up the sides of the neck to the base of the skull, applying pressure with your fingertips only. Make sure you do not apply pressure on the bony area of the neck nor anywhere near the throat. Repeat this effleurage stroke, breathing out on the downward stroke.

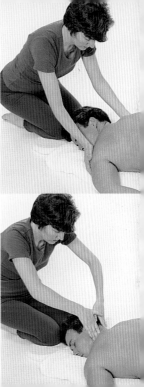

knuckle effleurage

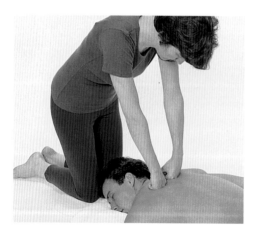

1. Clench your hands into fists with fingers pointing up toward you, knuckles on each side of the spine at the top of the back, 1½ inches apart. With great care, very slowly apply pressure with the flattest part of your fists and lean in, making sure this is comfortable for your partner.

2. With even pressure, take the fists down each side of the spine using the flat of the knuckles to apply pressure and keep your fingers pointing up toward you. The skin may turn red; this is quite normal and therapeutic providing your partner can tolerate it. The key is to work slowly.

3. Moving toward the lower back, flatten your hands just before reaching the lower back, glide them apart, and sweep one hand around toward each hip. Gently pull your hands back up as before in Steps 3–6, pages 167–169. Making sure your partner is comfortable at all times, you should be making tramline marks as you move down their back on each side of the spine. Try to keep even control and pressure on the downward stroke.

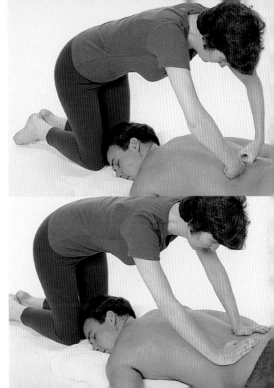

thumb effleurage

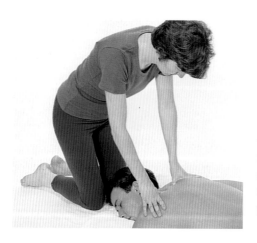

1. Place your thumbs on the top of the upper back on each side of the spine, about 1½ inches apart. Keep your fingers together but stretch them away from your thumbs. Make sure the flat pad of the thumb rather than the tip or nail is in contact with your partner.

2. Glide the thumbs with even pressure down each side of the spine toward the pelvis. You will need to be close to the spine to relax the muscles attached to it, which are responsible for spinal movement. Move slowly and evenly down the back, the fingers acting as guides to support the thumbs.

As you approach the lower back, sweep your hands apart toward the hips and glide your hands gently back up the sides of the back as before (see Steps 3–6, pages 167–169) ready to repeat the stroke.

3. You may notice specific areas of tightness as your thumbs travel down the back. Take a few seconds to apply static pressure with the thumb pads on these knots of tension. Gradually apply pressure to the area, going into the muscle slowly and leaning in with your body weight.

Hold for 5–10 seconds, then come away slowly. Check with your partner that you are not hurting them. After working on the tension knots, resume the thumb effleurage in Steps 1 and 2.

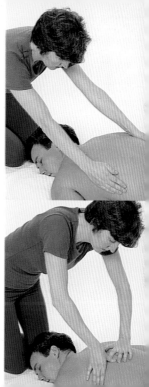

An aromatherapy massage is the perfect way to center yourself—to get back in touch with your inner core after being caught up in the rush and chaos of everyday events. The physical and mental serenity it creates will help you to reconnect with your own sense of values and to bring order and meaning to your day-to-day existence.

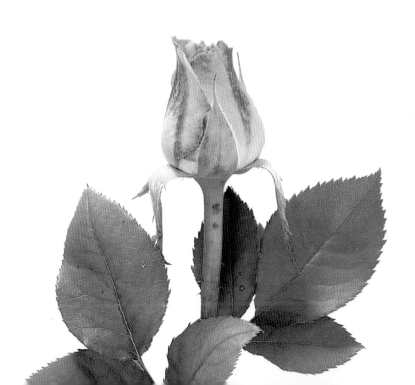

figure-eight

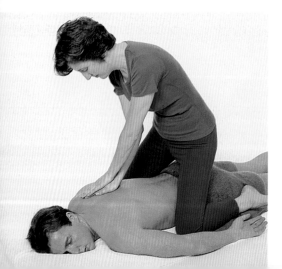

1. Position yourself by the side of your partner, making sure that you are comfortable. If you know the person well, you may feel more comfortable sitting astride them so you can work into both sides of the back with equal pressure and without putting strain on your own back.

Place one hand on top of the other and position both on the right side of the upper back with your fingers pointing toward the right shoulder. Firmly stroke over the shoulder with the flat of the bottom hand in a clockwise direction.

2. Glide over the shoulder joint, letting your fingers cup around the contours of their body, and apply firm pressure with the whole of the hand over the muscle that caps the shoulder joint and which you may see bulging in the upper arm. Pull this muscle firmly back toward you.

3. Lighten the pressure and continue the movement toward you, gliding your hand over the right shoulder blade and gently over the spine. Now point your fingers up toward the left shoulder and repeat the technique in Step 2, this time working in a counterclockwise direction. Make sure the complete movement forms a figure-eight over the entire upper back, flowing slowly and continuously.

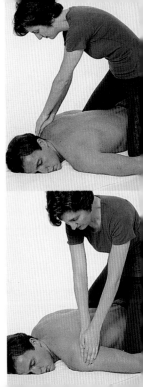

kneading the upper back

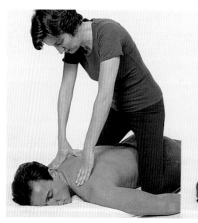
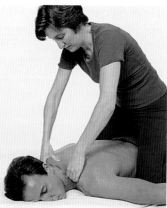

1. Place your hands on each side of the spine on the upper back, your fingers pointing forward and your thumbs stretched away from your fingers. Push the muscle on the top of the shoulder away from you and away from the bone, letting your thumbs "trail" gently behind.

2. Having your fingers close to the neck and away from the collarbone, trap as much muscle as you can between your fingers and thumbs, making sure it is not hurting your partner. Take care that your thumbs are not on their spine.

3. Using your fingers, pull the muscle toward your thumbs to manipulate the muscle and gradually let the bulk of the muscle "slip" from your fingers. Your thumbs will act as "anchors" to pull the muscle against, so try to keep them stationary, even though they may slip because of the oil.

4. Release the muscle and slide your hands outward ready to repeat the technique. Think of the complete action as a circular motion, circling in toward the neck, left hand clockwise and right hand counterclockwise. Begin each repetition by letting it flow from the end of the previous one.

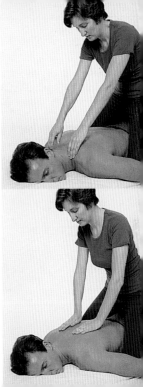

muscle-rolling

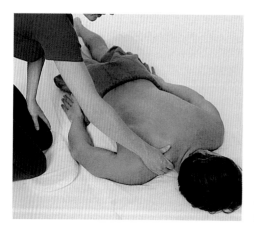

1. Position yourself on your partner's right side. Placing the fingers of your right hand on the top of your partner's right shoulder close to the neck, grasp the muscle firmly between the fingers and the thumb. Make sure you are manipulating muscle and not just skin, or you may pinch your partner during this movement. The more muscle you can pick up, the more effective the technique will be.

2. Keeping your fingers still, move your thumb toward your fingers, "rolling" the muscle until your thumb and fingers meet. Maintain the contact of your fingers with the top of the shoulder and repeat the rolling action with the thumbs. In this technique, you are literally grabbing the muscle and rolling, so once the initial contact has been made with the fingers, they remain in one spot and the thumbs create the movement. Repeat the rolling several times before moving on to the other shoulder to repeat the same sequence.

3. Muscle-rolling is relatively effortless and may be used as an alternative to kneading. On large muscles, you can roll both hands at the same time rather than alternately. Leaning forward as you roll your thumbs away from you will help the technique flow. Repeat on the other shoulder.

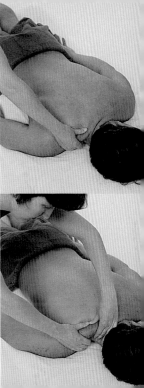

open-handed kneading

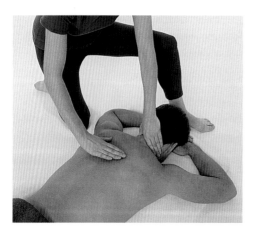

1. Position yourself at the left side of your partner, level with their neck, your head and shoulders facing them. You will need to adopt the half-kneeling position to be able to maximize the effectiveness of your body movement in this stroke. In order for your partner's neck to be straight, it may be necessary for them to place their hands, palms-down, under their forehead.

the neck

2. Placing the fingers of your left hand together and stretching your thumb away from them to form a "V," use the "V" to scoop the muscles on the top of the neck down toward the back. Work against the resistance offered by the strong muscle on the top of the shoulder. It is important to make sure pressure is applied evenly throughout the "V" of the hand during this stroke.

3. Repeat the action in the opposite direction with your right hand scooping up the neck muscle and into the hairline. Now repeat the whole movement. As one hand lifts off, the other takes over. Rock your body from side to side as your hands move in one direction and then the other.

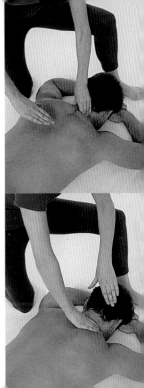

crisscross *This technique can be applied gently for a*

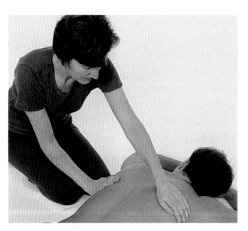

1. Position yourself facing your partner level with their chest. Place the flat of your hands, fingers and thumbs together, one on each side of the back starting at the top of the shoulders. Make sure both hands are pointing in the same direction away from you.

2. Pull your hands toward each other, lifting the muscle off the bone. For a strong manipulation, lift your body upward to help you. Cross your hands over the back so the one that started nearest to you becomes farthest away and vice versa. Try to keep as much of the palm of your hands as

relaxing massage or strongly to manipulate muscle.

possible in contact with your partner's skin as you crisscross your hands all the way down the back, avoiding any pressure on the spine.

3. On reaching the lower back, repeat several times up and then down the length of the back, finishing at the lower back.

Use an up-and-down motion of your body area. Keep the pace slow and try to establish a rhythm as you work down the back. Finish the back massage with an effleurage (see pages 164–169).

(see pages 164–169).

RECIPE FOR BACKACHE

2 drops rosemary oil,
1 drop sweet marjoram oil, and 1 drop ginger oil
Blend with 1½ tablespoons carrier oil.

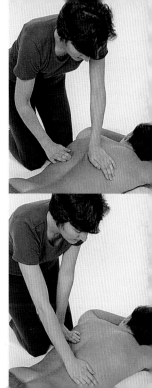

*M*assage is one of the oldest forms of healing. Its origins date back some 5,000 years to China. Both the ancient Greek and Roman civilizations used massage for relaxation and health. The most famous physician of all, Hippocrates, known as the "father of medicine," wrote in the 5th century B.C. that "the way to health is a scented bath and an oiled massage every day."

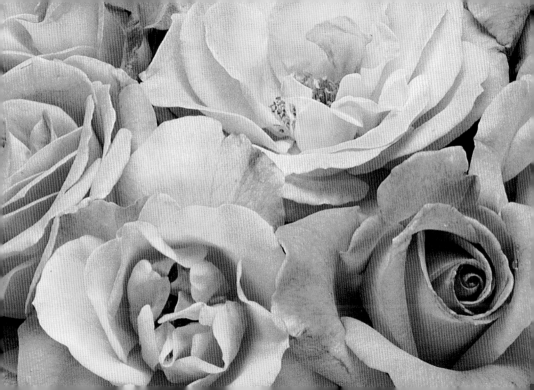

a complete foot massage

A foot massage can feel like the ultimate luxury. It is a truly relaxing massage and will help calm and rebalance the whole body through stimulation of the reflex points.

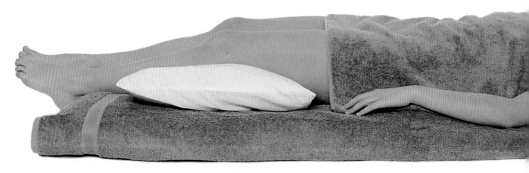

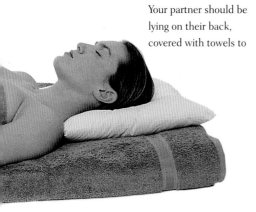

Your partner should be lying on their back, covered with towels to keep them thoroughly warm. Make sure they are absolutely comfortable—you may wish to put a pillow or rolled-up towel under their knees for extra support. Some people will need a pillow under their head. It is not advisable for heavily pregnant women to lie flat on their back, so prop them up with several pillows. Position yourself at the feet of your partner, and uncover one foot, keeping the rest of the leg covered for warmth. When performing a foot massage, remember to be very firm to avoid tickling your partner.

effleurage

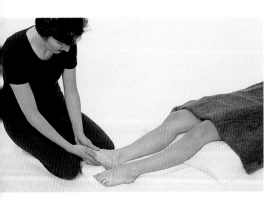

1. Position yourself facing the sole of your partner's exposed foot which you can turn slightly outward. Place your hands, one on the top and one on the sole of the foot, with your thumbs together along the side of the big toe. Your hands should be "sandwiching" the top and bottom of the foot ready to begin the effleurage.

2. Firmly slide both thumbs along the length of the instep toward the heel, keeping them parallel. Your fingers should be relaxed and trail behind the thumb in gentle support. This part of the foot represents the spine in reflexology terms, so this movement is particularly beneficial for lower back problems.

3. At the heel, slide your thumbs away from each other, around and back up each side of the instep toward the big toe. Apply pressure with your thumbs on the way down from toe to heel, with very little pressure on the return. Repeat 3 or 4 times.

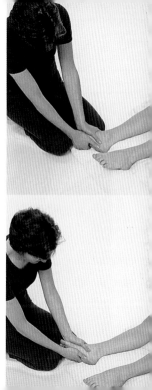

corkscrew

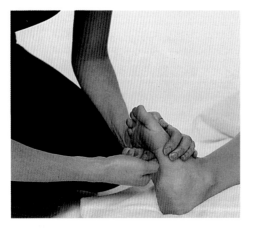

Supporting the top of the foot with one hand, make a fist with the other hand. Using the sharp edge of your knuckles, press into the sole of the foot while turning your wrist in one direction as far as it will go, in a corkscrew action. Then release and move your hand up the sole a little. Repeat this technique slowly all over the sole of the foot. You can use the hand supporting the top of the foot to push against.

rotating

1. Place one hand underneath the ankle, holding it firmly. With your other hand, take hold of your partner's foot by grasping the ball of the foot between fingers and thumb (keeping away from the toes if possible); make sure the whole of your hand is in contact with the body of the foot.

2. Lift the foot slightly off the floor with your hand supporting the ankle and using the other hand, begin to rotate the foot from the ankle slowly, working against its natural resistance. Gently increase the arc of the circle as much as the foot will allow, keeping a slow but constant pace.

Make 5 or 6 circles in one direction. Then repeat this action, rotating the foot in the opposite direction.

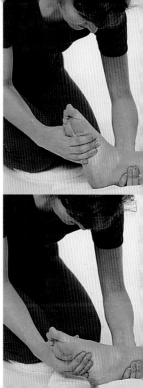

stretching

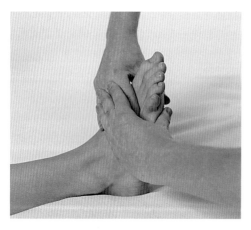

1. Place the thumbs overlapping on the ball of the foot and grasp the top of the foot with your fingers. Push your thumbs into the sole and at the same time pull your fingers down as if trying to pull the sides of the foot toward the center of the sole, exaggerating the arch of the foot. Work firmly against the resistance of the foot, taking care not to let your fingers or thumbs slide. Hold the stretch for 5–8 seconds and release slowly. You should be performing this stretch by going in and out of the movement slowly. On completion of this stretch, repeat several times, gradually moving your thumbs down toward the heel. You may be surprised at the amount of pressure your partner can withstand; feet are very strong and used to supporting a lot of weight and pressure all the time.

2. Once you have reached as far as you can going down the length of the foot, reverse the action by stretching the foot in the opposite direction, pushing the sides of the foot up and away from the center of the sole. Repeat slowly several times all the way back up toward the toes.

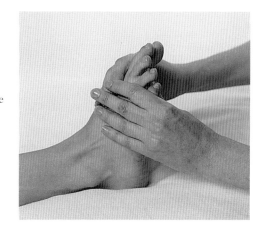

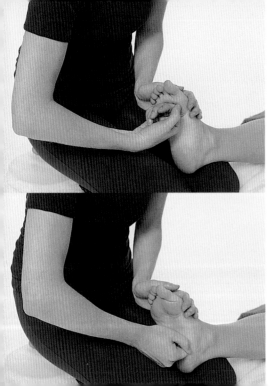

fist-stroking

1. Supporting the top of the foot with one hand, make a fist with the other hand. Turn your arm so the wrist is facing up. Stroke the sole of the foot from underneath the toes to the heel slowly with the flat of the fist, uncurling your wrist as you move downward.

2. Cover the full length of the sole of the foot. Repeat this technique 4 or 5 times, applying a little more pressure each time, always working downward and away from your body.

circular pressures

Grasp the top of the foot with the fingers of both hands and place the thumbs on the ball of the foot. Using the pads of the thumbs firmly, apply deep, slow, circular pressures, leaning in with your body weight on the initial part of the pressure to get depth into the muscle and circle outward away from an imaginary central line running down the length of the body. Your right thumb circles clockwise, your left counterclockwise. Once you have made several circular motions, lift the thumbs and place them a little farther down the sole. Repeat the technique covering the sole of the foot. Remember to keep at least one hand in contact with the foot at all times as you move between pressures. You can also perform this technique with one thumb only on each of the toes.

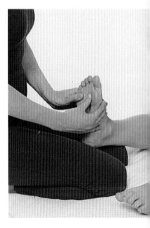

squeezing the toes

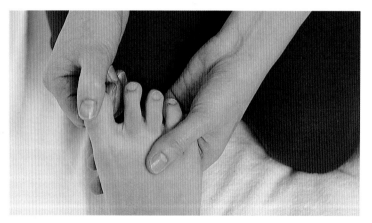

Support the foot with one hand and with the other squeeze each toe in turn from base to tip, between the fingers and thumb. Then gently pull and release. Grasping each toe between finger and thumb, you can also rotate each toe in turn to improve mobility.

lymph drainage

1. Being on your feet all day can result in swelling of the feet and ankles due to the accumulation of lymph, which is caused by gravity as well as poor circulation. This technique will help with the drainage of lymph back toward the heart. Working on the top of the foot, hold the toes down firmly with one thumb. This will cause the joints to open up.

2. Following the gaps between each of the toes one at a time, trace the spaces between the bones with the other thumb up toward the ankle. Stop when you reach the bridge of the foot. Lift the thumb off to repeat, working in each of the 4 spaces several times.

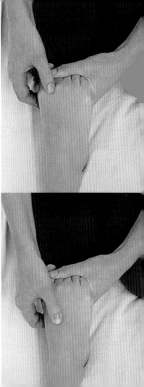

top-of-foot effleurage

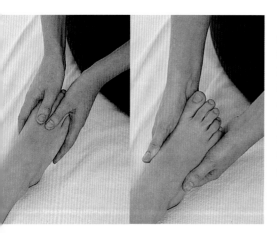

1. To continue to assist the drainage of lymph from your partner's lower limb, place your hands one on each side of the foot, with your thumbs on the top of the foot ready to begin to bring the foot massage to a close.

2. Firmly glide both thumbs up the center of the foot top toward the ankle, keeping them parallel. Relax and trail the fingers beside the thumb. Approaching the ankle, slide the thumbs away from each other, around and back down each side of the foot top toward the toes, ready to repeat the stroke.

stroking ankle joint

Place the fingertips of each hand each side of the ankle joint. Circle the fingers around the outsides of the prominent bone, slowly and gently. Sandwich the top and sole of the foot between your hands and slide them down toward the toes gently to finish the massage. Repeat the sequence on the other foot.

RECIPE TO SOOTHE ACHING FEET

1 drop peppermint oil and 1 drop rosemary oil
Blend with 2 teaspoons carrier oil.

Rosemary oil has warming properties.

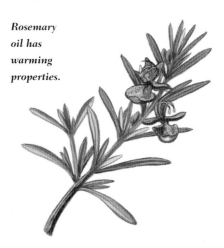

W hen blending oils with a carrier oil for massage, make up a favorite, beneficial recipe in a large batch for regular use. Store in dark, glass bottles with screw tops in a cool place away from sunlight. Remember to label and date, making a note of the combination of oils used and the quantities. They should keep in good condition for up to 16 weeks.

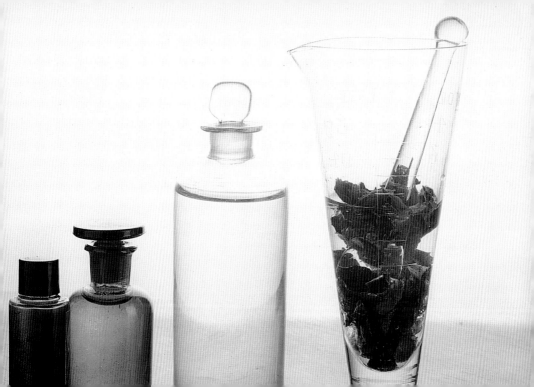

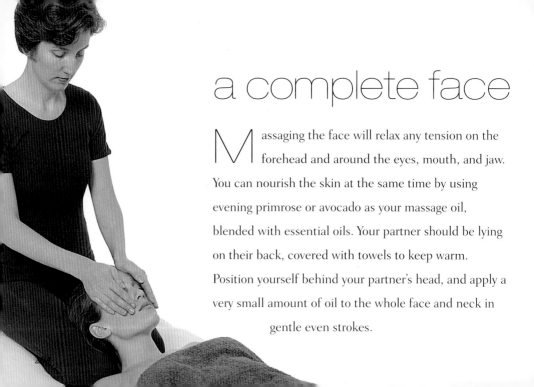

a complete face

Massaging the face will relax any tension on the forehead and around the eyes, mouth, and jaw. You can nourish the skin at the same time by using evening primrose or avocado as your massage oil, blended with essential oils. Your partner should be lying on their back, covered with towels to keep warm. Position yourself behind your partner's head, and apply a very small amount of oil to the whole face and neck in gentle even strokes.

massage

FACIAL RELAXATION
Cup your hands, fingers, and thumbs together, and place them gently over your partner's face, on each side of the nose. Encourage them to close their eyes and breathe slowly and deeply to relax. Hold this position for 20–30 seconds and use this time to relax yourself.

EFFLEURAGE
Place your hands, with the base of the thumbs touching, on your partner's forehead with your fingers cupping around the outer side of their temples. Stroke the base of the thumbs firmly outward across the forehead, the fingers gliding down the outer side of the face. Glide your hands all the way down the outer side until the fingers of both hands come together at the bottom of the chin. Glide your hands back up the sides of the face to meet, thumbs together, on the center of the forehead ready to repeat the effleurage.

Wheatgerm oil is also beneficial.

205

waterwheel effleurage

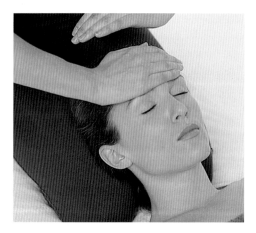

Continuing with another stroking technique, place one hand, fingers and thumb together, across the forehead, and this time stroke the whole hand back toward the hairline. Just as the first hand is about to lift off, the other hand repeats the action, so the hands are alternating in a circle above your partner's head, like the paddles of a waterwheel.

forehead effleurage

1. Place the heel of one hand on one side of your partner's forehead. With the wrist leading, and fingers and thumb together, stroke slowly and gently across the width of the forehead to the opposite side of your partner's head.

2. Just as the first hand is about to lift off, the other hand repeats the stroke in the opposite direction. Repeat this technique continuously, incorporating the rhythmical movements of your body with each stroke you make.

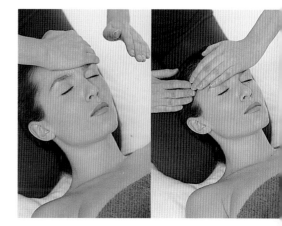

around the eyes

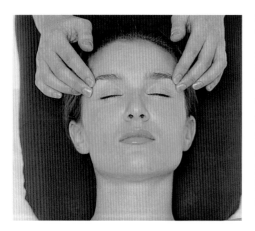

STROKING AROUND THE EYES

Following the direction of the eyebrow growth, begin to circle one or two fingers lightly around the complete eye area. Use the bone around the eye socket as your guide. Take care to be gentle and not to drag the delicate skin.

PRESSURE POINTS ON THE BROW-BONE

Using your index fingers, apply careful pressure underneath the brow-bone of each eye. Hold for a few seconds before gently lifting off the fingers. Repeat in 5 or 6 places as you move gradually outward across each brow-bone to the outer corner of each eye.

CIRCLING THE TEMPLES

Using the fingertips, gently find the very slight hollows of the temples on either side of the eyes. Maintaining full contact with the fingertips, begin to circle them slowly so that you feel the skin move with your fingertips, rather than making circles on the surface of the skin. This is a continuous movement with your fingertips remaining in the same position, and can be performed clockwise or anticlockwise.

RECIPE TO RELIEVE A HEADACHE

1 drop peppermint oil OR 1 drop lavender oil
Mix with 1 teaspoon carrier oil and rub a small amount into the temples.

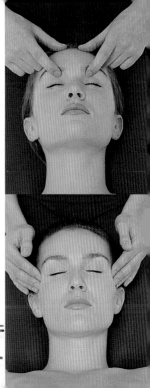

eyebrows and nose

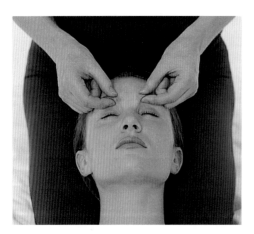

PINCHING THE EYEBROWS

Pinch each eyebrow between the index finger and thumb of each hand either side of the bridge of the nose. Hold for a few seconds before gently releasing. Repeat as you work outward. On reaching the end of the eyebrow, repeat the whole sequence.

STROKING THE NOSE

Place a thumb on each side of the bridge of your partner's nose with the fingers resting lightly on the outer sides of the face. Stroke down each side of the nose, lifting your thumbs off gently as you reach the nostrils, ready to repeat the action. This can help relieve blocked sinuses.

cheeks

STROKING THE CHEEKS

Keeping your hands lightly resting on the outer sides of the face, stroke the thumbs outward from each side of the nose across each cheek. Lift the thumbs just before they reach the ears and resume the movement, covering the whole cheek area.

PRESSURE POINTS ON THE SINUSES

Place the fingertips of each hand underneath each cheekbone and apply careful pressure upward into the bone. Gradually work your way along the length of each cheekbone in an outward direction. This may help to relieve the pain of blocked sinuses.

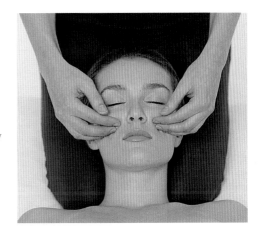

around the mouth

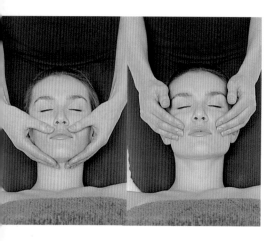

STROKING AROUND THE MOUTH
Again maintaining contact with the fingertips, stroke the thumbs across the skin above the top lip in an outward motion from the center of the face. As you reach the jawbone, lift your thumbs off gently and repeat the technique.

CIRCULAR PRESSURE ON THE CHEEKS
Using two or three fingertips of each hand, apply circular pressures all over the cheeks. This is particularly effective on the area where the upper and lower jaw meet, where tension can be held.

jaw

PINCHING THE JAW
Between the thumbs and curled index fingers of each hand, pinch the center of the chin and hold for a few seconds. Gently release the pressure and repeat, gradually following the line of the jaw outward. On reaching the outside of the jaw, work back in toward the chin.

SKIN-ROLLING
Using one hand, pinch the skin on the outside of one side of the jaw and roll your curled fingers very gently back toward you, pulling the skin of the jaw, keeping your thumb stationary. Repeat with the other hand and work with both hands alternately along the whole jawline from ear to ear. On reaching the other side, repeat the action in the opposite direction, but this time very gently roll your curled fingers away from you, pulling the skin of the jaw, keeping your thumb stationary.

Finish the massage with the effleurage sequence on page 205.

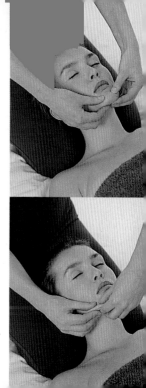

*F*or an ultimately relaxing full-body

massage, blend 3 drops of neroli oil

and 2 drops jasmine oil with 1½ tablespoons

carrier oil. Use long, soothing, and rhythmic

strokes (see pages 164–169)

with numerous repetitions over the whole body. Combine your aromatherapy massage with continuous, rhythmic instrumental music, for an ultra-sensuous experience.

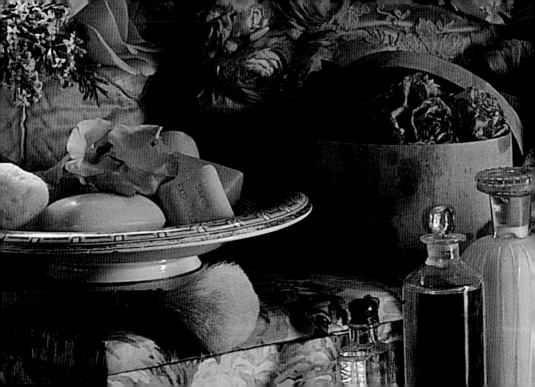

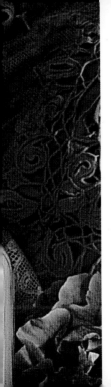

aromatic
interi🌸rs

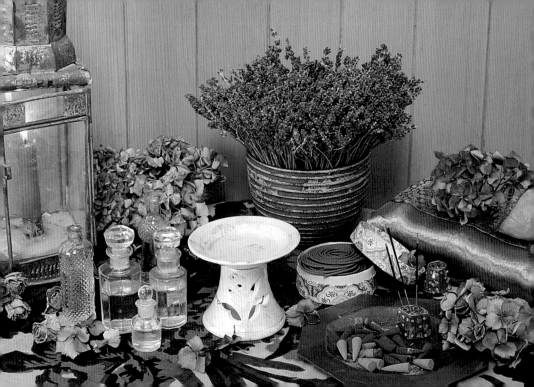

room vaporizers

The mood-enhancing and healing qualities of essential oils can be easily and effectively enjoyed as room fragrancers. Commercial essential oil burners are specially designed for this purpose, consisting of a small container, which should be filled with water and up to 5 drops of essential oil added (follow individual manufacturer's instructions), set over a votive candle. When the flame burns,

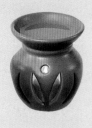

the oil is warmed and vaporized, dispersing the fragrance through the room. You can also purchase a special ring that surrounds a standard lightbulb and is designed to take a small quantity of essential oil. When the light is switched on, the heat from the bulb vaporizes the oil. Other ways of scenting a room and enjoying the effects of essential oils include misting the air with water from a pump-action spray to which 3 or 4 drops of oil have been added.

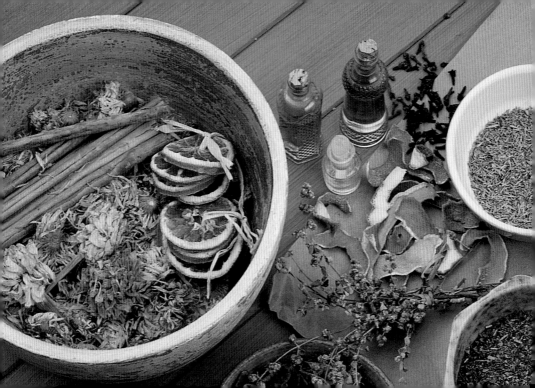

potpourri
with borage & bay

Make this colorful potpourri to place in decorative bowls around the home to fill the air with its spicy fragrance, or spoon the mixture into cheesecloth bags to scent clothes in drawers. In winter, put some of the potpourri in a dish and keep it by the fire where the warmth will release its aroma.

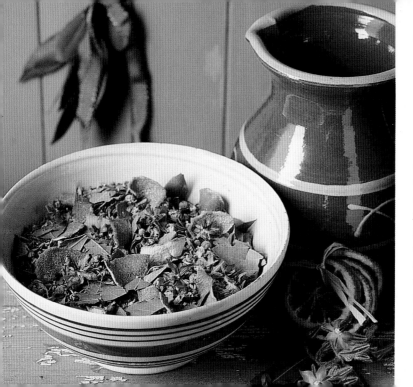

As an extra decoration, dry some borage flowers in silica gel to maintain their color and shape, and scatter them on the surface of the potpourri.

223

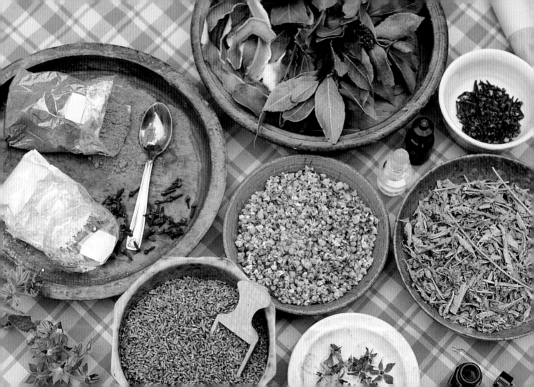

1/2 teaspoon grated
   nutmeg
1/2 teaspoon crushed
   cloves
2 tablespoons dried
   ground orris root
3 drops lavender oil
2 drops bay oil
1 drop rose geranium oil
1 cup dried lavender
   flowers
1 cup dried crumbled
   bayleaves

1 cup dried lemon
   verbena, lemon balm,
   or lemon thyme
1/2 cup dried chamomile
   flowers
1/2 cup dried borage
   flowers
1 teaspoon shredded
   dried orange rind

1. Put the spices in a bowl with the orris root and the essential oils and combine thoroughly as though rubbing fat into flour.

2. Mix together the dry ingredients, then stir in the spice mix. Place the potpourri in an airtight container. Store it for 6 weeks, shaking it from time to time, then decant into baskets.

rich rose
potpourri

The scents of the different layers of dried herbs in this special potpourri combine with time to give a delicious fragrance. Keep the potpourri for at least 6 weeks before use. Keeping it well sealed will improve the scent.

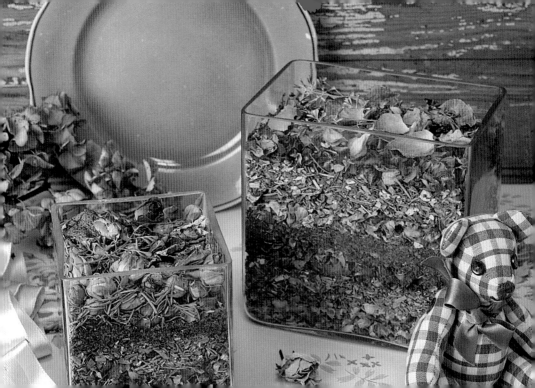

2½ cups dried pink and
red rose petals

2½ cups dried mint
leaves

4 tablespoons dried rue
sprigs

2½ cups dried red
rosebuds

4 tablespoons rosemary
flowers and leaves

¼ vanilla bean

2 tablespoons orris root

2 teaspoons ground
cinnamon

½ teaspoon ground
cloves

5 drops rose oil

5 drops rosemary oil

1 drop patchouli oil

1. Put the dried herbs into separate bowls. Chop the vanilla bean finely, then mix together the orris root, cinnamon, and cloves. Mix the oils together in a cup.

2. Put the dried herbs in a wide-mouthed jar in layers, starting with the rose petals, followed by a layer of mint, rue, rosebuds, and finally the rosemary. Over each layer, sprinkle a little of the orris, cinnamon, and clove mixture, and a drop or two of the oil mixture. Finish with a layer of rose petals.

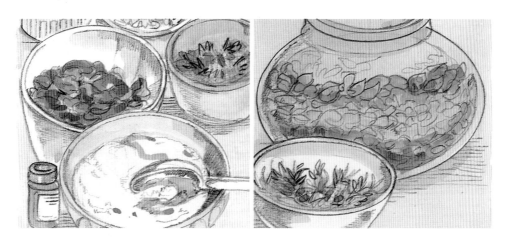

Tomorrow morning let a tent of colored brocade be raised . . . Fill it then with delicious perfumes of various kinds, amber, musk, and scented flowers such as the rose, orange-blossom, jonquil, jasmine, hyacinth, pink, and others similar. That done, you will place in the tent golden cassolettes filled with perfumes, such as green aloes, ambergris, nedde, and other pleasant odors. Then the tent must be closed that none of the perfume can escape . . . you will mount your throne and send for the prophetess . . . When she inhales the perfumes she will be delighted, all her joints will slacken, and she will swoon away.

The Perfumed Garden of Sheikh Nefzawi

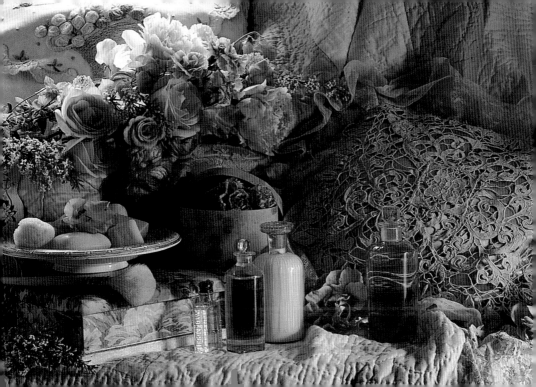

scented wooden shapes

Cedarwood essential oil is ideal for impregnating small wooden shapes to put inside drawers and closets, to scent their contents.

Cedarwood oil has a lovely spicy, resinous fragrance. Any plywood or light wooden shapes can be used—including those made out of cedarwood—or some of the carved and molded wooden objects specially designed to be used as scenters. Put the wooden shapes in a plastic bag, then sprinkle on the oil and shake the bag.

The fragrance can be topped up when needed by adding a few extra drops.

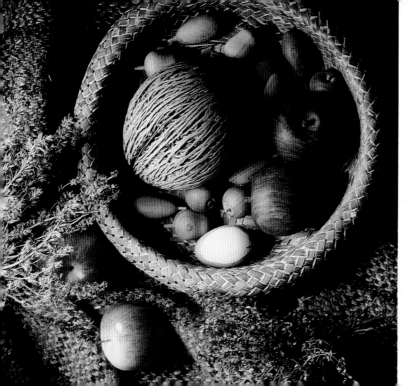

*Try using allspice
essential oil as a
more pungent
alternative to the
traditional cedar
fragrance for
impregnating
wooden shapes
and scenting
clothes.*

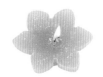

fragrant
candlelight

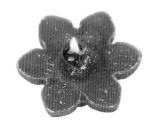

Y ou can make a simple yet effective fragrant candle using any suitable container into which you pour liquid wax. Empty seashells are ideal. The wick must be the right thickness for the diameter of the candle, or it may not burn properly. It is sold in long lengths, usually with instructions as to what size candle to use.

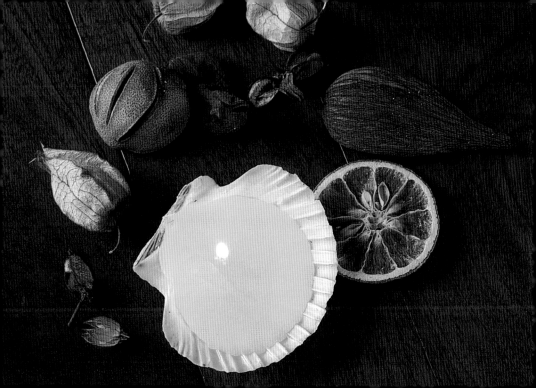

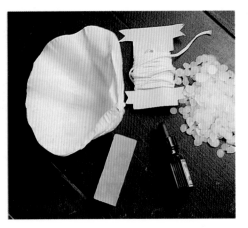

1. Choose an essential oil to scent your candles—rose, jasmine, citrus, vanilla, bergamot (oswego or bee-balm), ylang ylang, or citronella for outdoor candles. Use easy-to-melt plain, white candle wax granules and a small proportion of beeswax. Select clean shells that will stand flat on a surface.

2. Put the wax granules and beeswax in a small saucepan and melt it over a very low heat. Be very careful if your stove uses natural gas, since wax is flammable. Dip a length of wick into the melted wax and let it cool. This will make it stiff enough to insert into the shell.

3. Attach the wick to the base of the shell with a small piece of clay. Support the top of the wick with a wooden skewer. Add a few drops of essential oil to the melted wax, then pour carefully into the shell. Let it cool completely, then remove the skewer and trim the wick to $1/2$ inch in length.

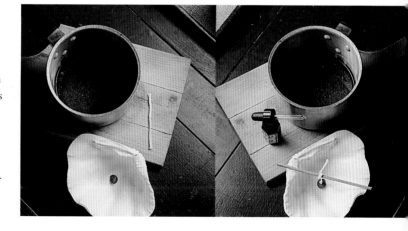

floating scenterpiece

A bowl of scented floating candles and fresh flowerheads makes a very elegant and atmospheric centerpiece for a dinner party or celebration. Buy small floating candles in a floral scent of your choice and in colors to coordinate with the flowers. Use brightly colored candles to complement boldly colored flowers, such as nasturtiums. Fill a decorative glass bowl about halfway with water and carefully float the flowers and candles on the surface, covering the whole surface of the water. The candles will not burn for very long, so do not light them until your guests are seated around the table. Use fragrant green herb leaves mixed with marigold or borage flowers as an alternative to nasturtiums, or scented full-blown roses.

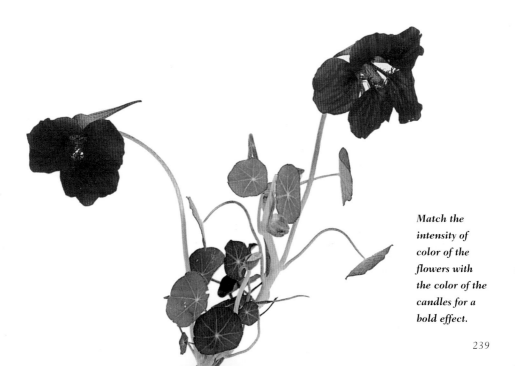

Match the intensity of color of the flowers with the color of the candles for a bold effect.

239

The tremulous and quivering sheen
Of their soft pinions white
I catch through rosy, golden tints
Which gleam from blossoms bright,
Their footsteps fall as noiselessly
As rose leaves from the stem,

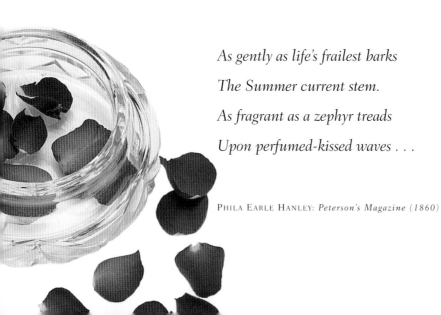

As gently as life's frailest barks

The Summer current stem.

As fragrant as a zephyr treads

Upon perfumed-kissed waves . . .

PHILA EARLE HANLEY: *Peterson's Magazine* (1860)

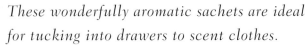

sweet powder
sachets

These wonderfully aromatic sachets are ideal for tucking into drawers to scent clothes.

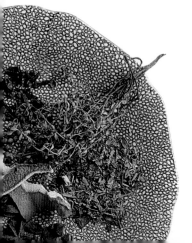

A lternatively, sew a pocket on a pillow and insert a sachet to impregnate the pillow with its fragrance. You need a spice- or coffee-grinder to make the sweet powder successfully, though you could buy the spices ready ground and crumble the larger leaves.

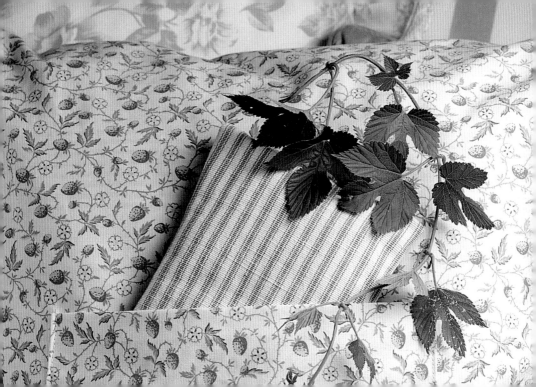

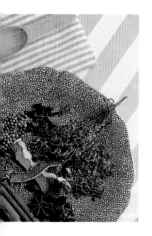

½ *cup dried thyme*
½ *cup dried rosemary*
½ *cup dried sweet*
  woodruff
1 *cup cinnamon sticks*
1 *cup dried orange peel*
½ *cup cloves*
½ *cup coriander seeds*
¼ *cup star anise*
¼ *cup powdered orris*
  root

1. You will need to make small bags with fairly wide-necked openings to hold the finished mixture. Strip the leaves from the stems of the thyme and other herbs.

2. Grind small batches of the mixture at a time, and empty the contents of the grinder container into a bowl after each grinding. Stir the finished mixture well, to distribute all the ingredients evenly. Scoop small amounts into the empty bags, and then sew or tie them to close.

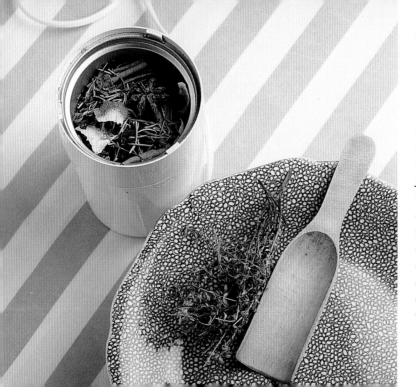

Dried orange peel is easy to make. Save any peel from oranges you have eaten and dry in a warm, dry place outdoors away from bright sunlight in summer, or over a heat source in winter.

245

aromatic fire bundles

Never throw away the stalks of lavender when you prune or trim your plants. Stack them in bundles and throw them on an open fire for a heady, perfumed smoke. They work well in wood-burning stoves, too. Store the fire bundles in the dark away from sunlight, which might otherwise leach out the perfumed oils in the stems.

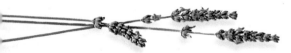

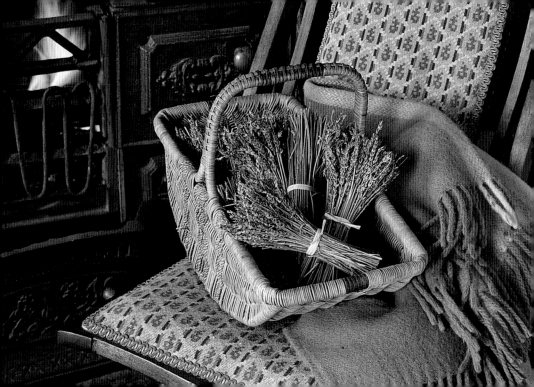

aromatic mats

Enjoy the delightfully comforting and appetizing aroma of lemon or lavender as you set a hot pan or teapot down on the kitchen table with these easy-to-make, herb-filled quilted place mats. Collect attractive fabric remnants to make them from, choosing a plain or contrasting patterned fabric for the backing and binding.

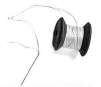

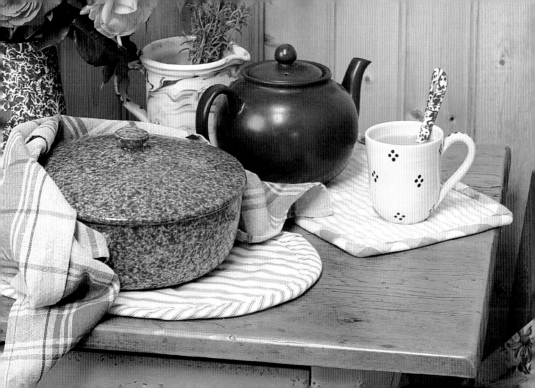

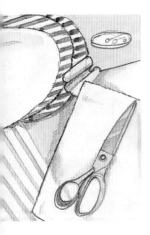

a piece of decorative fabric (8 x 11 inches for each mat)

a piece of backing fabric the same size

a piece of thin batting the same size

dried lavender or lemongrass

a length of bias binding (about 40 inches long for each mat)

dressmaking chalk

1. Measure and cut out the rectangle from the decorative fabric, backing fabric, and batting. (Round off the short sides for an oval-shaped mat.) Sew them together around the edge, leaving a section open for the herb stuffing. Draw guidelines for quilting in chalk on one side of the mat. Fill the mat with a good handful of the dried lavender or lemongrass. Sew up the opening by hand.

2. Keeping the mat flat so the stuffing does not shift, quilt the mat carefully by hand, or machine stitch along the chalk lines.

3. Pin, then stitch the bias binding to the edges of the mat.

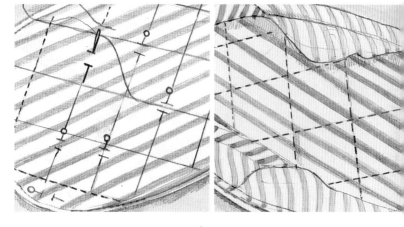

lavender
sleep toys

*Children will adore these
lavender-scented sleep toys to tuck
under their pillows at night.
They are simple to make and are
ideal stocking-fillers at Christmas.*

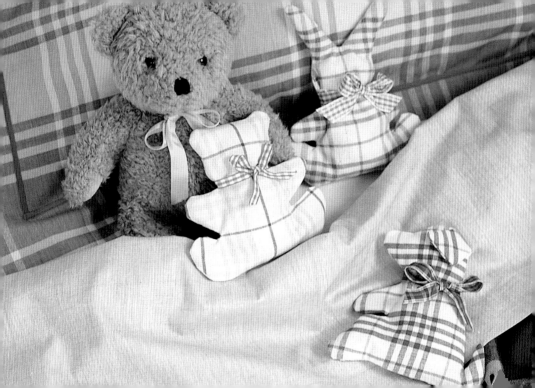

*scraps of brightly
  colored, patterned fabric*
*simple paper animal
  shapes, such as tedd
  bears and cats*
dried lavender flowers
*dressmaking chalk or
  felt-tip pen*
*yarn, braids, or
  decorative ribbon, for
  trimming*

1. Lay the animal shapes on the fabric and draw around them with the chalk or pen, allowing 3/8 inch all around for a seam allowance.

2. With right sides together, sew around the shape, leaving a section open at the bottom for the stuffing.

3. Turn the shape right side out, and stuff firmly with lavender, using a knitting needle to push the herb into the corners.

4. Sew up the opening. Add a tail made from lengths of braid or yarn, if appropriate, or trim with decorative ribbon tied in a bow.

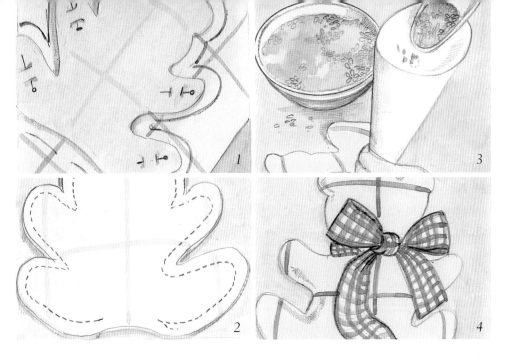

Let's go to that house, for the linen looks white, and smells of lavender, and I long to lie in a pair of sheets that smell so.

IZAAK WALTON: *The Compleat Angler* (1653)

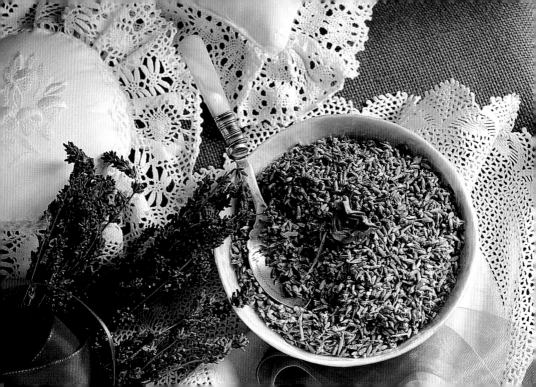

posies
of fragrance

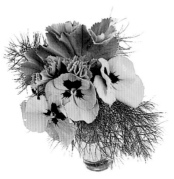

The tradition of making "tussiemussies"—posies of aromatic herbs and scented flowers—dates back to the Middle Ages, when they were carried by judges and other dignitaries to sweeten the air. You can also enjoy the sights and scents of flowers and foliage gathered from the garden, or even from a windowbox, by composing your own colorful, fragrant posies for displaying in vases.

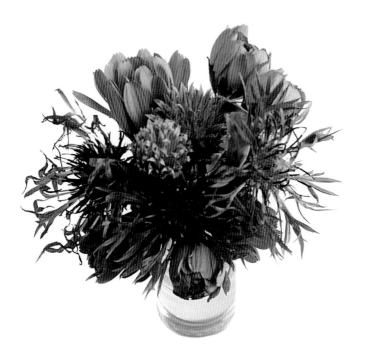

Taking color contrast to its limits, this posy is composed of deep blue bachelor's buttons, chive flowers with their delicately savory aroma, and sungold marigolds.

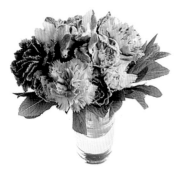

Try variegated mint, one of the prettiest and most aromatic of herbs, surrounded by coral, pink, and salmon garden pinks (*Dianthus* sp.) and an outer ring of fresh green garden mint (see left).

Lady's mantle (*alchemilla mollis*) leaves have the delightful habit of harboring dewdrops long after other plant material has dried. In the posy on page 258, the leaves and tightly furled buds are ringed around with yellow pansies fringed with feathery, aromatic fennel.

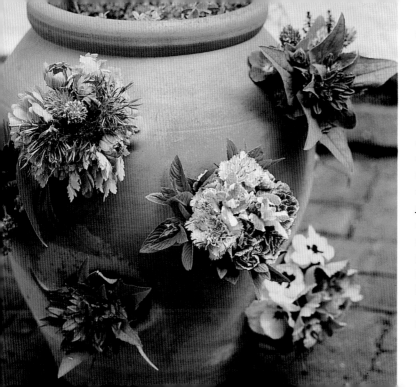

Alternatively, you could make a stunning special-occasion display of fragrant posies in a traditional terracotta herb pot. Set the stems in small plastic bags of water, tied at the top, to keep them fresh.

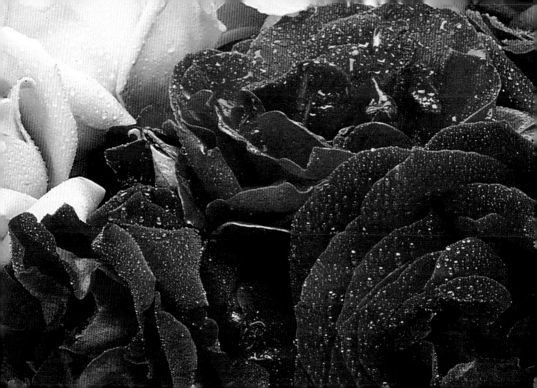

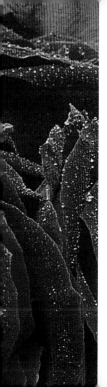

body
fragrance

scented soaps

Luxuriate in natural fragrance every time you bathe with these beautifying soaps, made to traditional recipes.

LAVENDER FLOWER
SOAP
*10 tablespoons grated
castile or pure soap*
*1 tablespoon Scented
and Citrus Honey
made with lavender
flowers (see page 370)*

*1 tablespoon Lavender
and Rosemary Flower
Water (see right)*
*2 tablespoons lavender
flowers, pounded*

For the Lavender and
Rosemary Flower Water
*4 tablespoons lavender
flowers*
*4 tablespoons rosemary
flowers or crumbled
rosemary leaves*
1 1/4 cups distilled water

1. To make the flower
water, put all the
ingredients in a small
enamel or flameproof
glass pan, cover, and
bring slowly to a boil.
Remove from the heat
and leave the infusion

for 1 hour. Strain away the flowers and leaves, pressing them against the strainer. Pour the liquid into a bottle, label it, and close it with a stopper.

2. Melt the soap and honey in the flower water in the top of a double boiler over simmering water. Remove from the heat, add the crushed lavender flowers,

and form the soap into balls. Place them on nonstick baking paper and leave in a warm, dry place for 2 weeks.

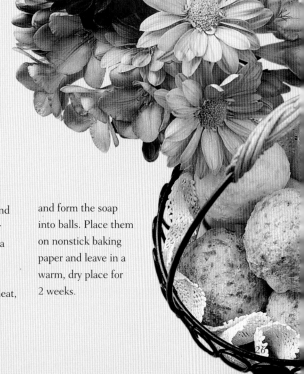

Oatmeal and Scented Honey Soap

10 tablespoons grated castile or pure soap

2 tablespoons water

1/2 teaspoon walnut oil

1 tablespoon Scented and Citrus Honey (see page 370)

2 tablespoons raw oatmeal, soaked and squeezed dry

1. Melt the grated soap in the water in a flameproof bowl over a pan of simmering water, or in a microwaveproof container in a microwave at the lowest setting. Stir in the walnut oil, 1 or 2 drops at a time, then stir in the honey and, when it has been absorbed, the oatmeal. Stir well and set aside to cool.

2. Shape the soap into balls and place them on a baking sheet lined with nonstick baking paper. Leave in a warm, dry place until the soap has set hard; this may take up to 2 weeks. When the soap has set, polish it with a clean, soft cloth and carefully smooth any rough edges.

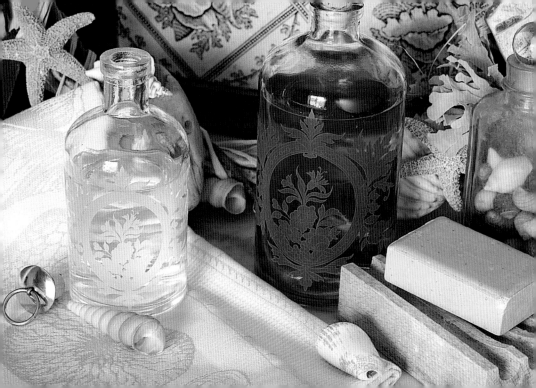

thyme bath bags

Aromatic herbs can be used to make a refreshing bath, which can soothe the skin and relax aching muscles.

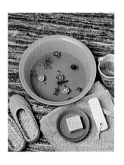

sprigs of fresh or dried thyme
8-inch square of cheesecloth
raw oatmeal (optional)
twine or ribbon

1. Break or crumble the thyme sprigs into small pieces and place in the center of the cheesecloth square. If you want to soften the bathwater as well, add a little raw oatmeal.

2. Gather together the corners and edges of the cheesecloth around the herbs and tie with twine or ribbon.

3. The bag can be hung from the faucet, left to float in the water as the bathtub fills, or used to scrub the skin.

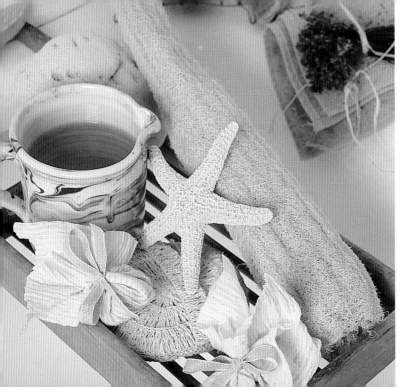

A simple way to enjoy a herbal bath is to make a strong infusion of aromatic herbs of your choice, strain them, then pour the liquid directly into the bathwater.

269

The barge she sat in, like a burnished throne,

Burned on the water; the poop was beaten gold,

Purple the sails, and so perfumed, that

The winds were love-sick with them . . .

. . . A seeming mermaid steers; the silken tackle

Swell with the touches of those flower-soft hands . . .

WILLIAM SHAKESPEARE: *Antony and Cleopatra* (1606–07)

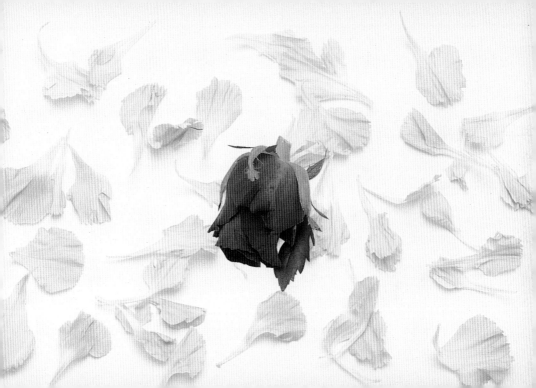

herb
bubble-bath gel

This recipe makes a lovely silky bath to soak in, with an invigorating scent provided by the fresh herbs and the lemon verbena essential oil. Pour the gel into the bathtub before running the water to create a nice foam. Castile or pure soap for making the gel can be bought from pharmacies.

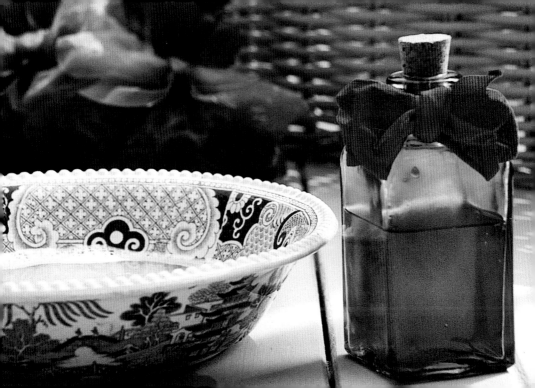

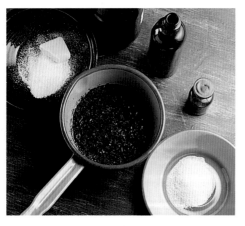

1 tablespoon sweet
woodruff
1 tablespoon mint
1 tablespoon comfrey
1 tablespoon angelica
5 tablespoons castile
or pure soap
2 tablespoons glycerine
2 teaspoons witch hazel
5 drops lemon verbena
oil
1 tablespoon unflavored
gelatin

*Makes about 1 1/2 cups
gel*

1. Measure out the
ingredients. Bring 1 cup
water to a boil and make
an infusion of the herbs
and the boiling water.
Grate the soap.

2. Strain the infusion and discard the herbs. Add the soap, stirring well. Combine the glycerine and witch hazel, then add the essential oil. Add this to the herb mixture.

3. When everything is thoroughly mixed, add the gelatin and stir until it is completely dissolved. When cool, transfer the mixture to small screw-top jars or glass bottles with cork stoppers.

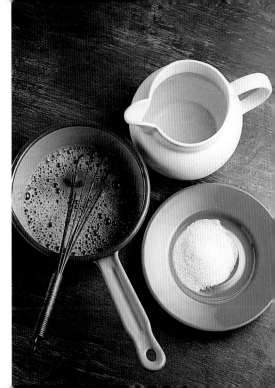

aromatic bath oils

Bath oils work by settling a film of oil over the surface of the water—they do not disperse in the water unless they are in an emulsion. They leave the skin feeling very soft and, with the addition of essential oils, wonderfully perfumed. Pat your skin dry after the bath rather than rubbing it.

1/2 cup tincture of benzoin
1/4 cup avocado oil
10 drops sandalwood oil
10 drops cinnamon oil
10 drops orange oil
10 drops basil oil
10 drops rosemary oil

Combine all the ingredients in a screw-top jar and shake thoroughly to mix. Use 1 tablespoon per bath. You can use almond or apricot oil in place of avocado oil.

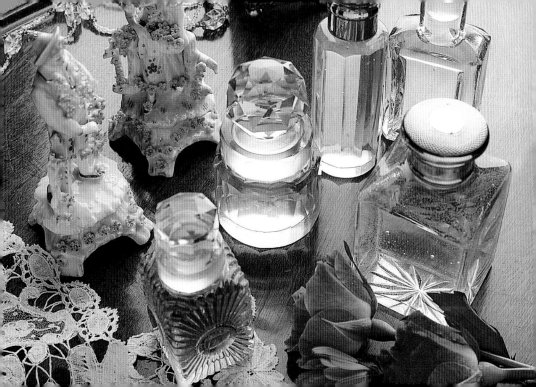

flower
waters

Herbs have been used throughout history to make fragrant waters to freshen and scent the body. Rosemary flowers and roses macerated in alcohol are the basic ingredients of Hungary Water, an ancient perfume. It was invented in 1370 by a hermit for the 72-year-old Dionna Izabella, the Queen of Hungary.

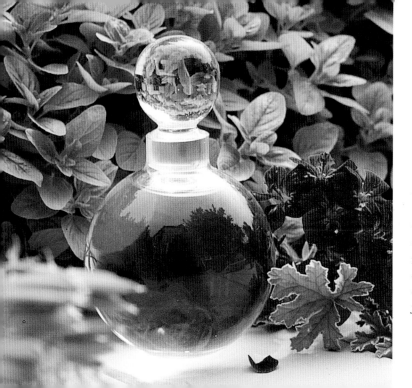

True rosewater is the gently fragrant byproduct of the distillation process by which the essential oil is extracted from the petals. It may be added to bathwater or to rinsing water for the hair.

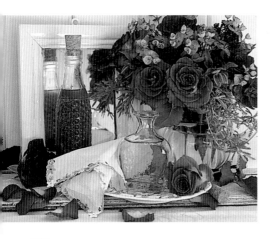

Hungary Water

4 tablespoons rosemary

4 tablespoons scented
   rose petals

4 tablespoons mint

2 tablespoons grated
   lemon rind

1 1/4 cups rosewater

1 1/4 cups orangeflower
   water

1 1/4 cups vodka

Makes 3 3/4 cups

1. Pound the rosemary leaves with the rose petals and mint. Add the grated lemon rind. Transfer to a wide-mouthed jar and cover with the rosewater, orangeflower water, and vodka.

2. Leave to steep for 2 weeks, then strain into a bottle and seal tightly.

Leave to mature for 1 month before using.

EAU-DE-COLOGNE
This classic scent also has a long history, dating back to the 18th century. Its sharp, citrusy fragrance is very refreshing.

4 tablespoons bergamot
    leaves or 10 drops
    bergamot oil
8 tablespoons rosemary
    leaves
grated rind of 1 orange
grated rind of 1 lemon
3 drops neroli oil
1 1/2 cups vodka

Makes 1 1/2 cups

1. Put all the ingredients in a wide-mouthed jar and cover with the vodka. Leave to macerate for 3 weeks, shaking the jar from time to time.

2. Strain into a clean bottle and leave for at least 2 weeks to mature.

Traditionally, eau-de-cologne contains bergamot leaves, from an orangelike tree, but if you cannot find these, bergamot oil can be used instead.

rose & vanilla
perfume

This is a rich, sweet perfume that is very feminine and delicious. Rose oil is an expensive essential oil, so you can substitute rose geranium oil for a cheaper alternative. When using vanilla for cosmetics, always use the pure oil or extract, never the alcohol-based extract used in cooking.

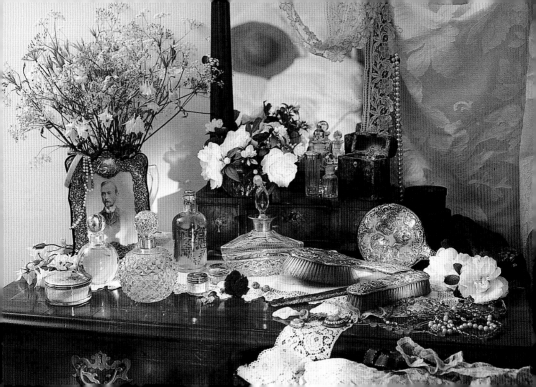

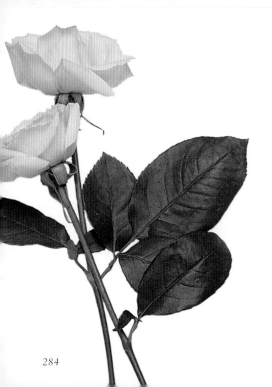

1/3 *cup vodka*
1 *cup scented dried rose*
  petals
2 *vanilla beans*
1 *tablespoon rosewater*
10 *drops rose oil*
10 *drops vanilla oil*
10 *drops petitgrain oil*
5 *drops ylang ylang oil*

1. Put the vodka and rose petals in a glass container. Slightly crush the vanilla beans and steep with the rose petals in the vodka. Cover and leave for about 1 week.

2. Strain the vodka, then add the rosewater. Stir thoroughly.

3. Add the drops of essential oils, stirring constantly. Bottle the

liquid and leave to mature for about 4 weeks. Strain the perfume once more through a filter paper and bottle before using.

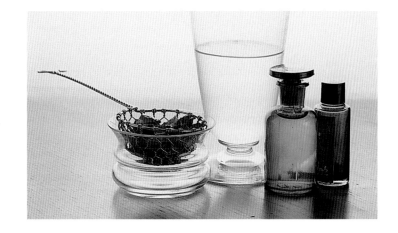

walnut, bay, & balm
footbath

This footbath will do wonders for tired, aching feet. Make a strong infusion of fresh herbs by steeping about 9 cups of herbs in 1 quart of boiling water. Include the following: English walnut leaves, bay, rosemary, lavender, sage, and lemon balm. You can use the leaves of butternut, black walnut, pecan, or wintergreen (checkerberry) in place of English walnut. Strain the liquid and whisk in 1 tablespoon of castile or pure soap to 1 quart of infusion. Add a few drops of rosemary and bay oils, and soak the feet in it for at least 10 minutes. Pat them dry.

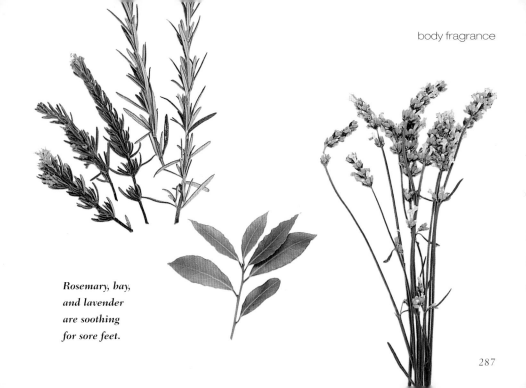

*Rosemary, bay,
and lavender
are soothing
for sore feet.*

287

lime
skin freshner for men

This citrus-based, spicy-scented, splash-on cologne can be used all over the body as well as on the face. The limes must be as fresh as possible, or the oils in the skins will have evaporated. Tincture of benzoin is added to act as both a preservative and an astringent.

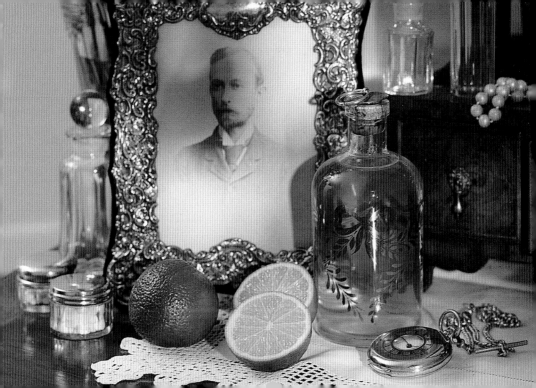

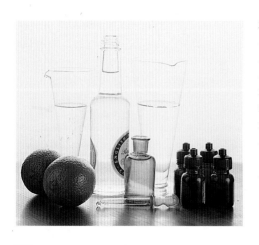

2 *fresh limes*
1 *cup vodka*
15 *drops lime oil*
10 *drops petitgrain oil*
5 *drops lavender oil*
5 *drops bergamot oil*
5 *drops bayleaf oil*
1 *teaspoon tincture of*
  benzoin
1 *cup rosewater*

1. Gather together all the ingredients and put to one side, except for the vodka and limes. Measure out the vodka.

2. Peel the limes and put the peel into the vodka. Cover and leave to steep for a week.

3. Put the drops of essential oil and the

benzoin into the rosewater and stir thoroughly. Strain the vodka and discard the lime peel. Mix the rosewater with the vodka, stir well, and bottle. Leave for 4 weeks. Strain again through a paper filter, then bottle finally before use.

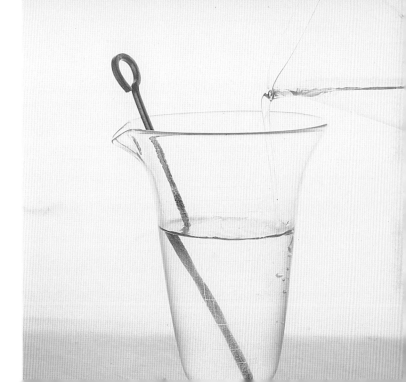

Once you have tried mixing and making your own fragrances, you may find that you wish to experiment further, creating your own personal perfumes. These unique handmade scents will also make very special gifts for friends and family. Look out for decorative bottles in which to store and package your creations, but remember that they must have a completely airtight stopper to prevent the contents from evaporating.

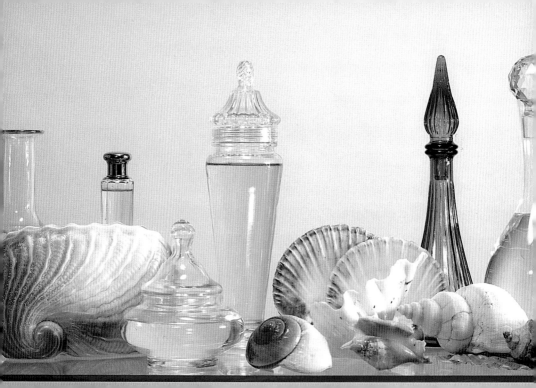

rose
steam treatment

One of the simplest of all beauty treatments is a herbal steam bath, to open the pores and deep-cleanse the skin, with the added bonus of scented herbs to soothe and heal. Simply mix a handful or two of fresh or dried herbs of your choice in a bowl of very hot water. Let them infuse for a few seconds, then put your face over them and cover your head with a towel to keep the heat in. Highly scented roses picked from the garden in summer make the most delicious treatment. Alternatively, try basil, chamomile, or a combination of fennel and lavender.

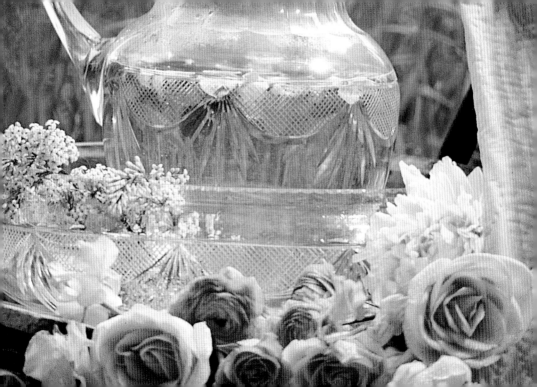

mint cleanser

This wonderfully aromatic cleanser is cooling and soothing on the skin. You can make it in a blender if you prefer, but rinse the face well after use to remove any shreds of mint. Sprinkle it on a cotton ball and rub it over your skin instead of soap. It is particularly good for delicate skin.

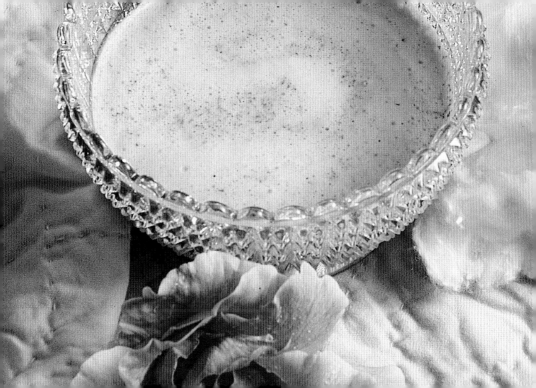

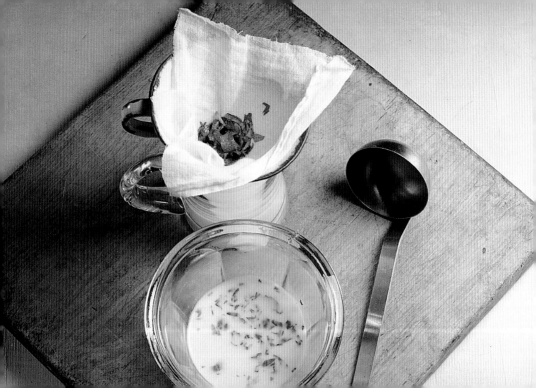

2 1/4 *cups fresh milk*
4 *tablespoons fresh mint*
(apple, eau-de-cologne,
or peppermint)

1. Measure the milk
and pour it into a clean
bowl. Wash and dry the
mint.

2. Chop the mint finely,
and add it to the milk.
Leave to infuse
in the refrigerator for
about 12 hours.

3. Strain the liquid
and bottle it. Store it
in the refrigerator.

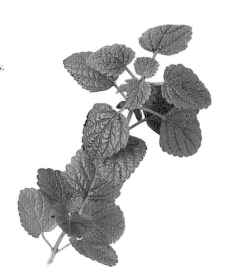

apricot & orange
moisturizer

This is a fairly rich cream for replenishing the skin with a warm and luxurious fragrance. Orangeflower water is good for dry skin and stimulates cell replacement. If you want to tint the cream, use a tiny amount of natural food coloring to make it a pale apricot color.

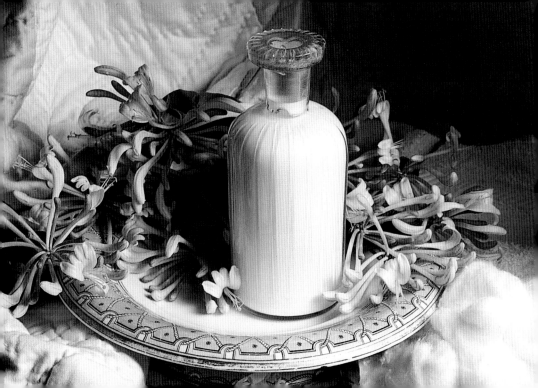

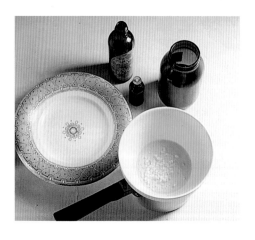

2 teaspoons white
  beeswax granules
4 tablespoons apricot
  kernel oil
2 tablespoons coconut
  oil
2 tablespoons glycerine
2 tablespoons
  orangeflower water
3 drops orange oil

1. Melt the beeswax
and apricot kernel and
coconut oils in the top
half of a double boiler,
over hot water, stirring
until they are
completely dissolved.

2. Add the glycerine to
the beeswax and oils,
and stir thoroughly.
Warm the orangeflower
water separately.

3. Remove the double boiler from the heat and add the orange-flower water, drop by drop, beating all the time, until it is a smooth cream. Add the orange oil and stir well. Add food coloring if you wish. Put into small screw-top jars.

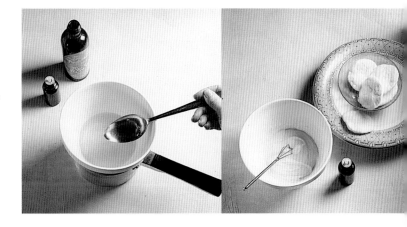

Besides bathing in asses' milk, Cleopatra liked to perfume her bathwater and scent her body with essence of rose. Rose essential oil was also used to make the first cold cream ever invented, by the Greek physician Galen in the 2nd century.

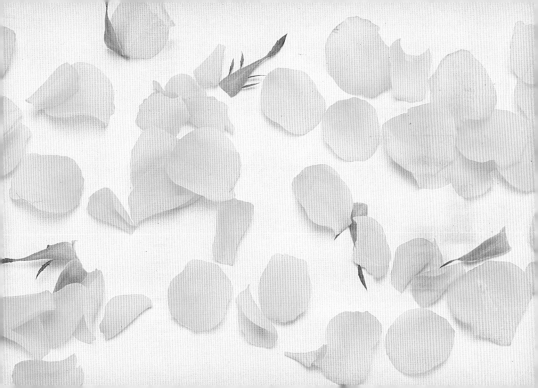

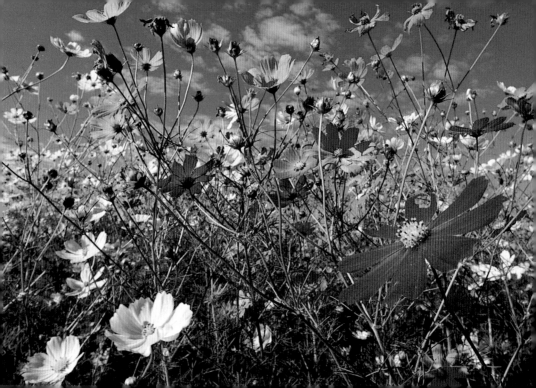

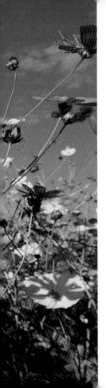

outdoor aromas

the influences of outdoor

The creation of a restful yet stimulating outdoor environment, full of interesting fragrances, encourages the healing process. Minds relax, but are also kept active and responsive by the wide range of aromas that plants can offer. Some scents from plants, such as honey, resin, and musklike fragrances, are warm and reassuring, while others with fruity redolences resembling raspberries, apples, and pineapples are the

scent

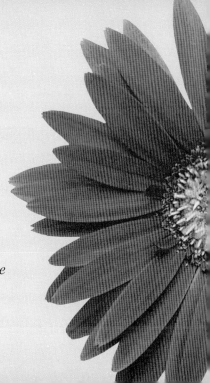

epitome of summer and slightly more stimulating. However, the comforting powers of scent are not always a result of the pleasantness of a particular smell but because the fragrance is especially evocative and triggers fond memories.

fragrant flowers

Sweet and heavily scented:

A universally comforting and pleasing perfume type. Classic flowering favorites in this category are the Madonna Lily (*Lilium candidum*), some daphnes, Lily of the Valley (*Convallaria majalis*), Mock Orange (*Philadelphus coronarius*), lilac, and viburnums.

Aromatic: These flowers contain the same oils found in many leaves, such as vanilla, balsam, and almond.

Plants in this group are native to many areas throughout the world, and include the Korean shrub *Virburnum carlesii*, Chinese Witch

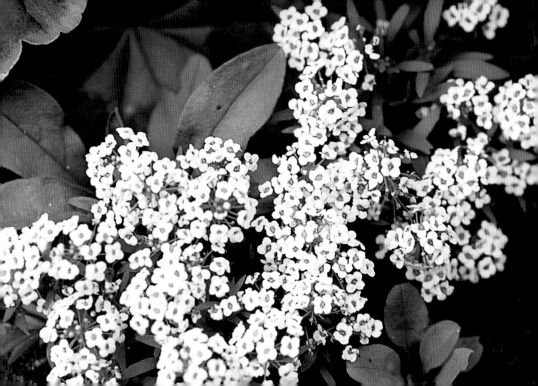

Hazel (*Hamamelis mollis*), Mexican Orange Blossom (*Choisya ternata*), and *Clematis flammula* from Southern Europe.

Honey: A fragrance found in many flowers including those of the common edging plant Sweet Alyssum (*Lobularia maritima*) and the diminutively bulbous *Crocus chrysanthus*.

Violet: A subtle fragrance that reveals itself one moment, then suddenly disappears only to reappear later. In addition to the many violets, this group includes the delicate and bulbous *Iris reticulata*, *Crinum x powellii*, several mimosas, and the Snowflake, *Leucojum vernum*, from central Europe.

Sweet and fruity: In addition to the many roses (see pages 332–335 and pages 340–343), flowers in this scent category include the Tree

Peony (*Paeony suffruticosa*), some magnolias, gorse, the Moroccan treelike shrub *Cytisus battandieri*, and the Beardless Iris (*Iris graminea*). Lemon is easily detected in the Macartney Rose of China (*Rosa bracteata*) and the North American Yellow Sand Verbena (*Abronia latifolia*).

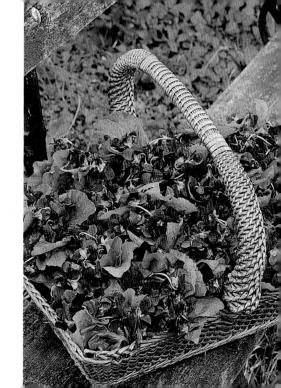

T o bring true calm to your mind and body, find a comfortable place to lie down in quiet solitude having picked a single, scented flower or sprig of herb whose fragrance you particularly like. Lay it down beside you so that you can breathe in its heady scent. Focus your mind entirely on the perfume and nothing else while you let the minutes glide by, letting it flow into and around your body to envelope it in its soothing vapors.

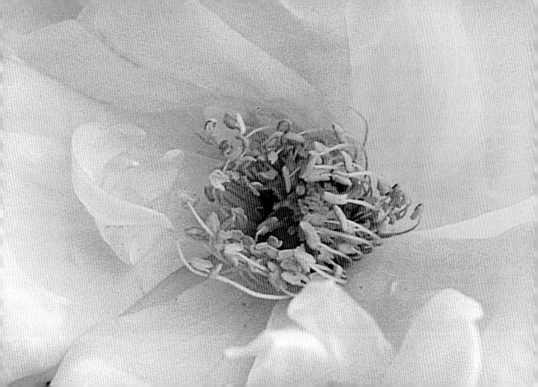

scented primulas

Primulas are highly attractive flowering plants, and many have a lovely fragrance. They thrive in moist soil, and are best planted in large groups, for maximum effect.

Primula beesiana develops whorls of fragrant, lilac-purple flowers on sturdy stems in summer.

The Drumstick Primrose, or *Primula*

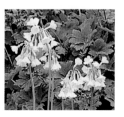

denticulata, is widely grown and has densely packed globular heads of lavender-blue flowers in spring and early summer. There are rose-purple and white forms, and they all have a wonderful honeylike scent.

The plant is not adapted to warm-winter regions, as with many primroses.

The Tibetan Primrose, *Primula florindae*, has sweetly scented, pale yellow, bell-shaped flowers during the summer, while *Primula prolifera* has fragrant golden-yellow flowers.

The Himalayan Cowslip, *Primula sikkimensis*, has delicately sweet perfumed, pale yellow flowers borne in pendant clusters during the summer months.

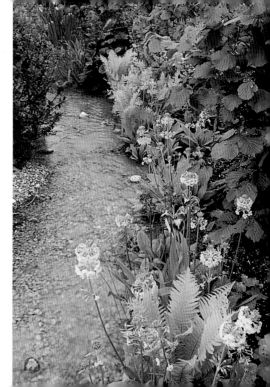

scented leaves

Turpentine: This stimulating fragrance type is best represented by the Southern European evergreen shrub rosemary, *Rosmarinus officinalis*.

Camphor and eucalyptus: There are several shrubs and trees that give off this distinctive and uplifting type of aroma, including the North American Carolina Allspice (*Calycanthus floridus*) and of course eucalyptus trees themselves.

Menthol: This essential oil is found in mint and some scented pelargoniums.

Sulfur: A category of savory aroma offered by garlic, onions, and mustard.

Flower: These scents are provided by the leaves of the Apple Geranium (*Pelargonium odoratissimum*) and the Sweet Briar Rose (*Rosa rubiginosa*).

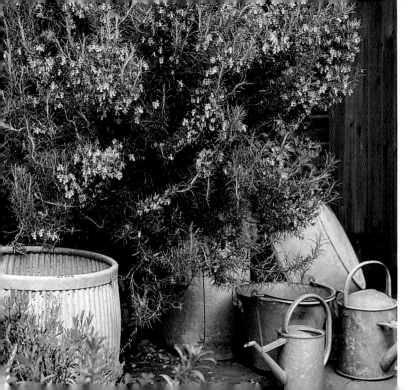

Rosemary has aromatic, needle-shaped, blue-green leaves, and produces blue, pink, or white flowers in late spring or mild weather. It grows well in a large pot or tub. Pinch out the growing points from all shoots in the first two years to keep the shrub low and bushy.

a boxful of scent

Scented pelargoniums are lovely, trouble-free plants to grow in a greenhouse, yard, patio, or garden. Each variety has a slightly different scent in its foliage, from apple and orange, to rose-lemon or peppermint. Many have quite insignificant flowers but are grown for their fragrant foliage. A fruit box provides an ideal, rough textured container for a collection of scented pelargoniums.

PLANTING AND MAINTENANCE

Line the fruit box with plastic and fill with good, gravely soil or packaged potting mixture. Plant a mixture of pelargoniums perhaps with a lavender or rosemary plant for foliage contrast and additional fragrance. Position the box in a sunny position, and water sparingly but regularly.

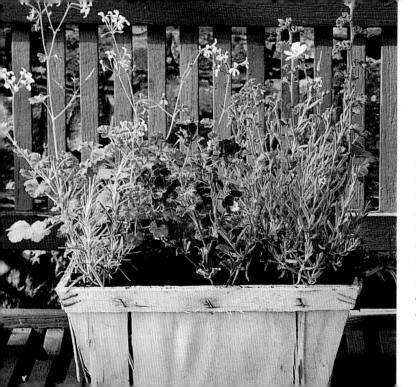

To make an attractive visual display, add a few more showy types of pelargoniums to the highly scented varieties, such as the Uniques or Regals, to provide a succession of colorful flowers.

a scented
boundary

A herbal hedge not only makes an aromatic edge to a herb garden.

Create a low-growing scented boundary to a flower border using herbs. Lavender is the ideal choice, with its attractive flowers and heady aroma. The quickest and easiest way of making a lavender hedge is to use

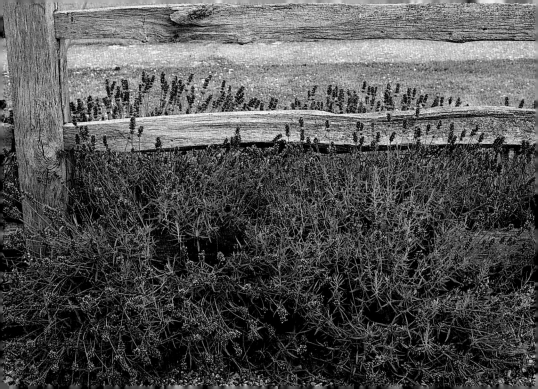

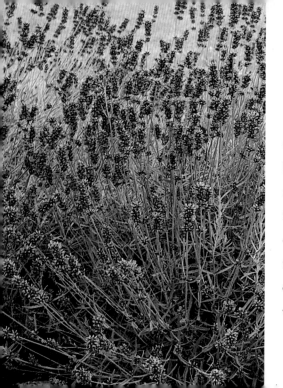

container-grown cuttings, either those you have taken yourself or bought from a nursery. Water the plants well in the first few weeks while they are becoming established. When they are fully grown, they will also need watering during periods of drought, because the thick bushy growth will stop moisture from reaching the roots.

1. Use a length of twine and 2 pegs to mark a straight line, or length of hose to make a curve, and make a row of holes where your plants are to go. Sprinkle a little organic fertilizer in and around the site.

2. Working as quickly as possible so that the roots are not exposed to the elements, set your plants into the ground. Full-size lavenders should be set 24 inches apart; smaller varieties, such as 'Munstead,' about 12 inches apart.

3. Clip the tops regularly to encourage side growth. Once the hedge is established, cut it back severely each spring. As it grows, trim the hedge so that the sides slope a little and the base is broader than the top.

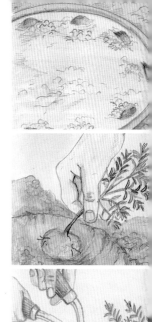

aromatic shrubs

Shrubs with aromatic leaves offer stimulating and unusual scents throughout the year, and are ideal for planting alongside pathways.

Lemon: The Lemon-scented Verbena, *Aloysia triphylla*, is a slightly tender deciduous shrub with pale to midgreen, lance-shaped leaves that have a strong lemon bouquet when crushed.

Orange: The Mexican Orange Bush, *Choisya ternata*, is a slightly tender, evergreen shrub with glossy, green leaves that yield the delightful fragrance of oranges when bruised.

Pungent: Rue or Herb of Grace, *Ruta graveolens*, is a well-known hardy, evergreen shrub with glaucous, bluish-green leaves and mustard-yellow flowers during mid and late summer.

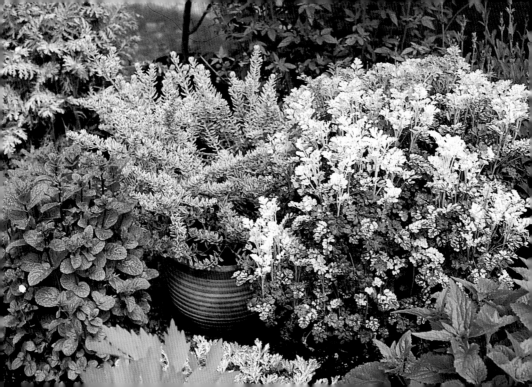

*T*was midnight—through the lattice wreath'd

With woodbine, many a perfume breath'd

From plants that wake while others sleep,

From timid jasmine buds, that keep

Their odour to themselves all day,

But when sunshine dies away,

Let the delicious secret out

To every breeze that roams about.

THOMAS MOORE (1779–1852)

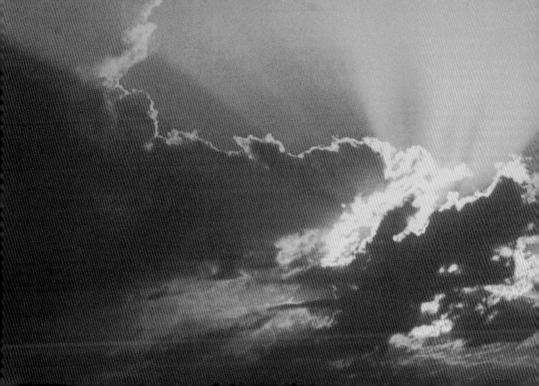

sweet evening fragrance

Most of the summer evening plant fragrances are sweet. The Sand Verbena (*Abronia fragrans*) is a half-hardy perennial with exceptionally sweet, pure-white flowers that open on summer afternoons. The Flowering Tobacco Plant or Jasmine Tobacco Plant (*Nicotiana alata*) is a half-hardy annual and

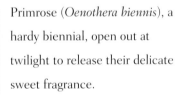

also has very sweet, tubular, white flowers. The pale yellow flowers of the Evening Primrose (*Oenothera biennis*), a hardy biennial, open out at twilight to release their delicate sweet fragrance.

Phlox paniculata, or Border Plox, is a herbaceous perennial with very sweet flowers borne in dense heads.

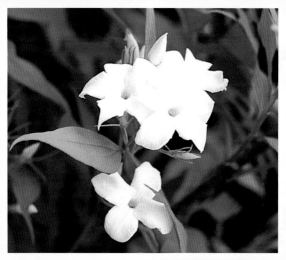

scented
roses

*The many types of fragrance
that these cherished shrubs
can offer range from the fresh
redolence of apples to the oriental
undertones of musk and the
fruitlike bouquet of bananas.*

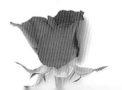

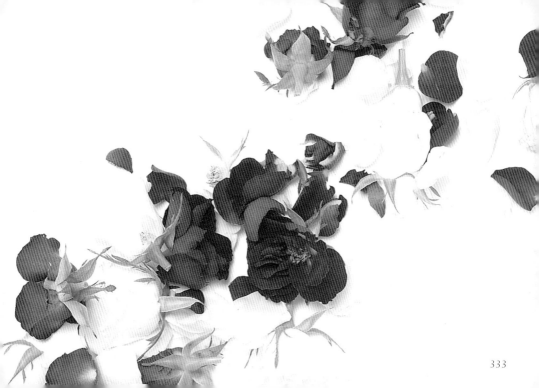

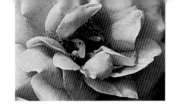

Apple: 'Max Graf' with its single, pink flowers has a shrubby nature and is ideal as ground cover. 'Nymphenburg' has apple-scented fully-double, warm salmon-pink flowers shaded cerise, with orange-yellow at the base of each petal.

Bananas: 'Dupontii' offers this unusual fragrance. It is a wild rose hybrid shrub with blush-white, cream-tinted flowers.

Lemon: A refreshing scent found in the large, double, white blooms of 'Mme Hardy,' a Damask type. The Hybrid Tea 'Blue Moon' has large, lilac-mauve blooms on upright, branching bushes, while the New English Rose 'Heritage' has medium-sized, cupped, shell-pink flowers.

Lilac: The Modern Shrub Rose 'Lavender Lassie' has this fragrance of early summer in its medium-sized, double, pink blooms shaded with lavender.

Musk: An essence of the East found in the deep-purple flowers of 'Cardinal Hume,' a New English Rose, as well as in the semidouble yellow flowers of 'Daybreak,' together with the large trusses of creamy-white flowers of 'Moonlight,' both Hybrid Musk roses.

Myrrh: 'Chaucer,' with rose-pink flowers, 'Cressida,' with large, apricot-pink flowers, and 'Cymbeline,' with loosely double, gray-pink flowers, all have this exotic fragrance.

Raspberry: A fresh, fruity bouquet found in the large, semidouble, rich pink flowers of 'Adam Messerich' and the pale-pink flowers, striped with crimson and mauve, of 'Honorine de Brabant.'

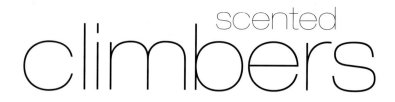

scented climbers

Sweetness is the kind of scent offered by most climbers,
but some have more exciting fragrances.

The ordinary Sweet Pea, *Lathyrus odoratus*, has a distinctive, heady redolence. It is a self-clinging, hardy annual with delicate pealike flowers in a wide range of colors, including pink,

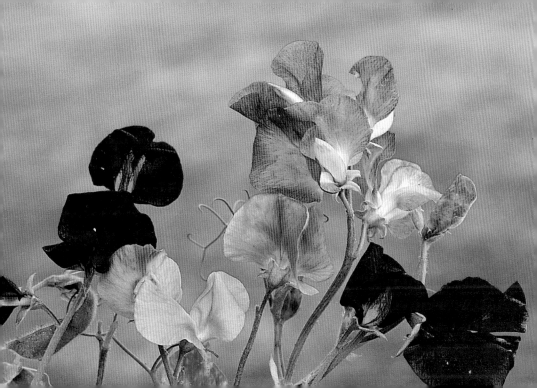

red, white, and purple, produced from mid summer to fall.

The flowers of the Common White Jasmine or Jassamine (*Jasminum officinale*) have a wonderfully rich, exotic scent which is slightly oriental in quality. It is a deciduous climber, with white flowers borne in clusters in the summer.

A honeylike fragrance is offered by the flowers of *Lonicera* x *americana*, a semievergreen or deciduous climber. The white or cream flowers become yellow and tinged purple on the outside during the summer. A related species, *Lonicera* x *heckrottii*, is hardy, deciduous, and with a shrublike habit. It bears yellow flowers flushed with purple of a similar scent during the summer.

Many honeysuckles offer a richly sweet fragrance with their delicate, eye-catching flowers. But they cannot hope to match the Blue Crown Passion Flower (*Passiflora caerulea*) for the sheer drama of its unusual and intricately designed blooms, which have a subtly sweet scent. It creates a superb display when planted against a sheltered, warm wall.

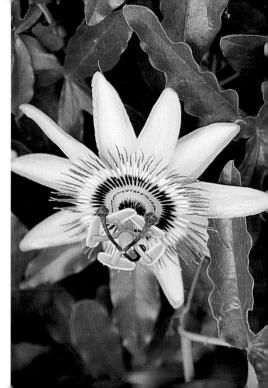

fragrant
rambling &
climbing
roses

In addition to drenching the air with sweetness, several roses that climb skyward have unusual bouquets to stimulate the senses and uplift the spirits.

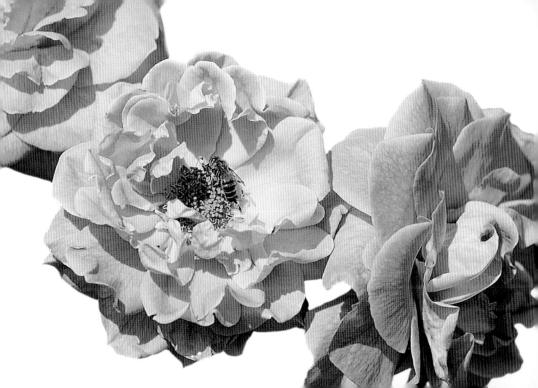

Ramblers have long, flexible stems, ideal for clothing arches and arbors, or rambling through trees. Climbers are ideal for growing against permanent frameworks on house walls.

Varieties with a fruity scent include 'Alberic Barbier,' a rambler with yellow buds that open to double, creamy-white flowers.

'New Dawn,' a climber, has silvery, blush-pink flowers that deepen toward the center.

'Francois Juranville' is a rambler with an applelike scent from its coral-pink flowers.

The unusual scent of myrrh is produced by the large, apricot-pink blooms of a New English Rose called 'Cressida.' The clear

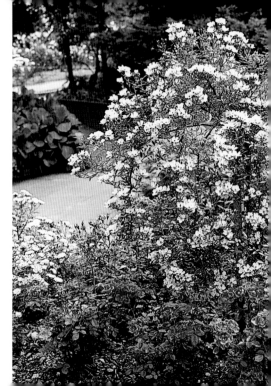

The rambler 'Felicité et Perpétue' has a delicate primroselike scent.

pink flowers of 'Constance Spry,' another well-known New English Rose, also have this distinctive bouquet.

Besides the Musk Rose (*Rosa moschata*), a climber with sprays of single, glistening white flowers, 'Aimée Vibert' offers an intoxicating musk fragrance with its graceful sprays of small, double, pure white flowers and yellow stamens.

I cannot see what flowers are at my feet,

Nor what soft incense hangs upon the boughs,

But in embalmed darkness, guess each sweet

Wherewith the seasonable month endows

The grass, the thicket, and the fruit-tree wild;

White hawthorn, and the pastoral eglantine;

Fast-fading violets cover'd up in leaves;

And mid-May's eldest child,

The coming musk-rose, full of dewy wine,

The murmurous haunt of flies on summer eves.

JOHN KEATS (1795–1821): *Ode to a Nightingale*

pots of
aroma

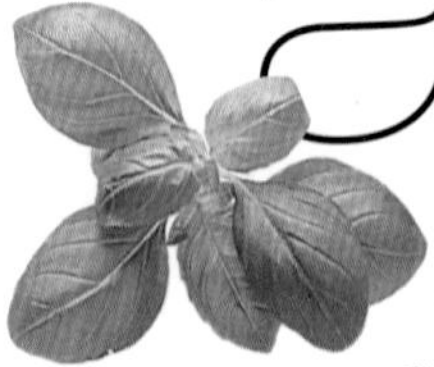

*Herbs offer
an abundance
of scent to stimulate
the senses and
soothe the mind.*

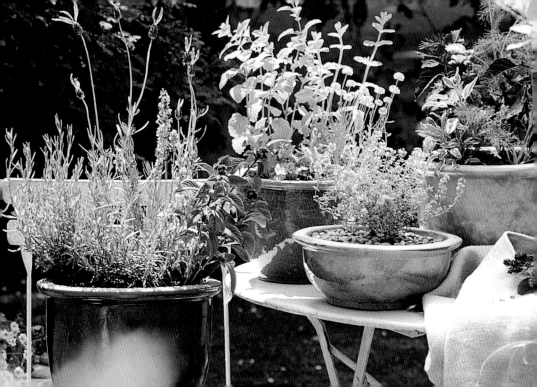

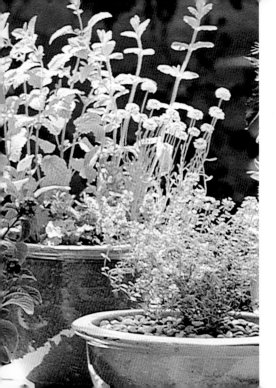

Highly practical and versatile, scented herbs can be dried and used to make scented sachets and potpourris, while culinary varieties add fragrant flavor to a wide variety of drinks and dishes. Growing herbs in containers allows even the smallest city yard or patio to enjoy their special aromatic qualities. Bringing them

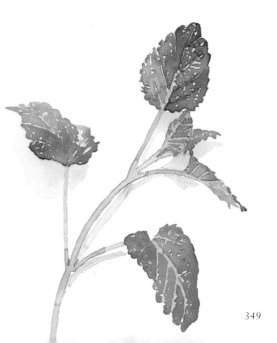

up above ground level, too, means that you are tempted to pinch a leaf as you pass, or release the scent as you brush against the plants. It is important when mixing herbs together in a container to choose those that require similar growing conditions, in terms of the amount of sunlight and moisture needed.

golden-leafed fragrance

This container planting of golden-leafed herbs will keep its fresh color throughout the summer. Stand it out of the sunlight to help keep the colors fresh. Golden-leafed herbs prefer shade or semishade. Lemon balm both tastes and smells of lemon, and its aromatic scent attracts bees. It bears pale yellow or white flowers in summer.

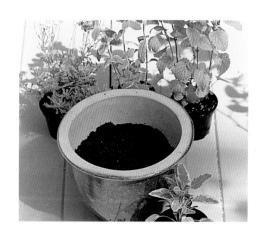

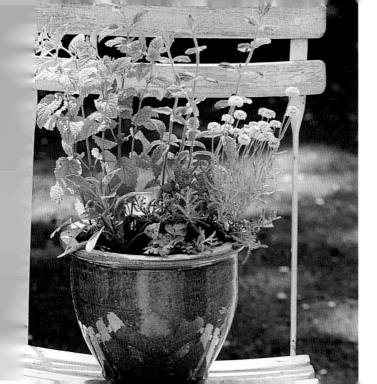

*1 tall ceramic pot,
2 golden lemon balm
plants,1 lemon-flowered
santolina, 1 cream
variegated sage*

Put pieces of broken
terracotta flowerpot in
the base of the
container for drainage.
Fill with a good soil-
based potting mixture.
Plant the two balms at
the back, the santolina
on one side, and the
sage on the other. Fill
with more soil if
necessary. Water well.

351

mediterranean medley

L avender is a fragrant herb of Mediterranean origin, and blooming fields of lavender found in the south of France are a breathtaking sight. There are many different varieties to choose from. In this planting, French lavender is combined with dwarf English lavender and purple-flowered heliotrope (*Heliotropium peruviana*)—sometimes called cherry pie because of its scent. Use a well-drained soil or potting mixture and, at the end of the summer, move the pot into a greenhouse or shelter it from frost in some other way. This combination of aromatic plants is especially good for a sunny site. Replace the heliotrope each year, or try using other herbs combined with the lavenders.

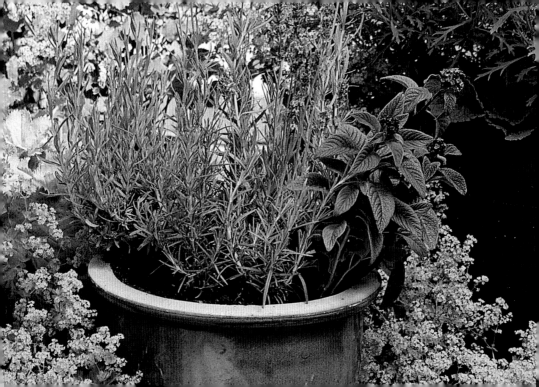

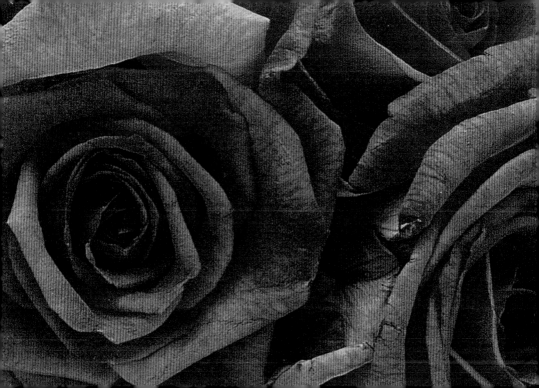

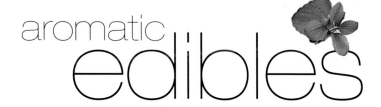

aromatic edibles

herb tea trio

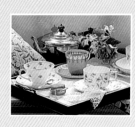

Herb teas have long histories as medicinal cures. They can soothe, calm, or invigorate, depending on the particular herb used. Chamomile tisane is a good relaxant; rose-petal tea is a refreshing, delicately fragrant drink; and jasmine tea is highly scented and goes well with strong and spicy foods, or after a meal. Make jasmine tea the same way as rose-

petal tea (see page 358), but use half
the quantity of dried flowers. To make
chamomile tisane, use a teaspoonful of
the dried flowers per person in a small teapot
and pour in just-boiled water, or use an infuser
and a teaspoonful of the herb to make a single cup.

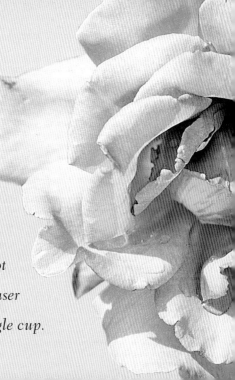

rose-petal tea

Rose-petal and other flower-flavored teas, as with most China teas, are meant to be drunk without milk. They are suitable for drinking with sweet foods, or as the perfect accompaniment to Chinese or other oriental meals.

2 tablespoons scented dried rose petals (pink or red)

1/2 cup black China tea leaves (such as Oolong)

If the roses are whole, dried heads, strip off the petals and use just the largest outside ones. Measure the tea. Scatter the petals over the tea leaves and stir them together. Pack in suitable containers for storing, or to make gifts. Little wooden or cardboard gift boxes are ideal for the purpose.

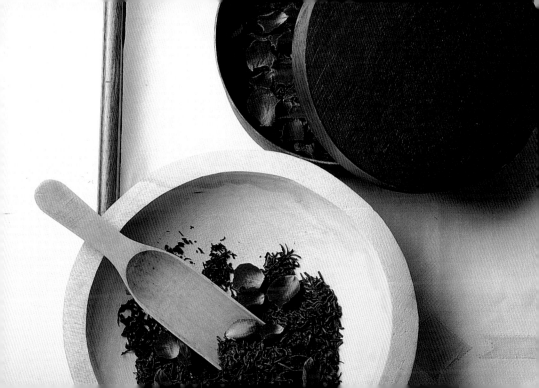

mint tea

This is a classic herb tea, full of refreshing fragrant flavor. The best mint to use is Moroccan mint (*Mentha viridis*). Failing that, use peppermint, which is a good aid to digestion. Moroccans sometimes add sweet marjoram to the mint in winter.

1 1/2 tablespoons green tea (available from specialist tea suppliers)
handful of whole fresh mint leaves
1/4 cup lump sugar

1. Rinse a teapot with boiling water. Put in the tea and cover with the mint. Add the sugar and fill the teapot with boiling water.

2. Leave to draw for 5 minutes, taking care that the mint does not rise above the surface of the water. Pour into small glasses. In Morocco, they make two pots of tea at a time and pour the liquid from both pots into the glasses simultaneously.

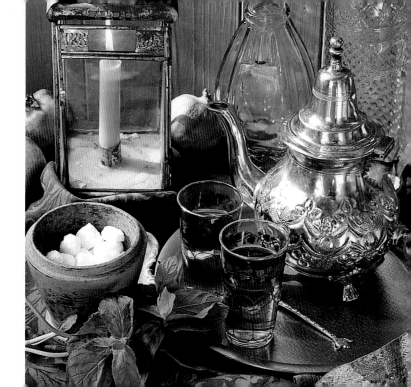

Herbal teas and tisanes offer the perfect way to unwind and relieve fatigue after a hard day's work, to replenish both the mind and the body. Take the opportunity, when elderflowers are in blossom, to make a tisane from them. Use about 1 tablespoon of the fresh blooms per cup, and let them infuse in boiling water for several minutes. The tisane is gently reviving with a beautiful, soothing fragrance—a lovely way to bring your day to a close.

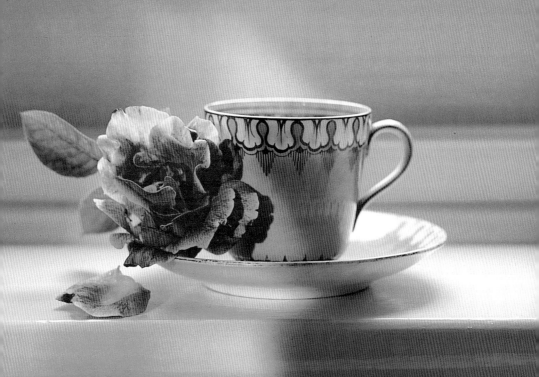

scented
flower cordials & syrups

*Capture the uplifting scents of
summer flowers in concentrated syrups and
cordials, then release their sweetly fragrant
flavor in tall, refreshing drinks
made with sparkling water and crushed
ice, or in fruit salads, or drizzled over
ice cream and sherbet.*

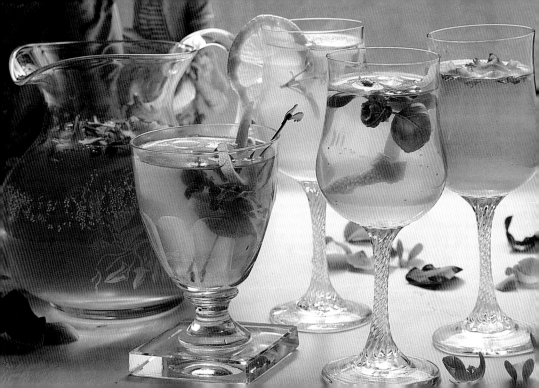

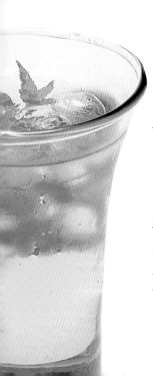

JASMINE CORDIAL
1 cup jasmine flowers
1 cup superfine sugar
1 pint boiling water

1. Make layers of the jasmine flowers and sugar in a glass or china bowl, cover, and set aside for several hours or overnight.

2. Pour in the boiling water, stir well, cover, and leave for about 8 hours.

3. Strain the liquid into a pan through a nylon strainer, pressing the flowers against the sides to extract as much flavor as possible.

4. Bring the liquid to a boil and boil it rapidly for 10 minutes or until it becomes syrupy. Leave it to cool slightly, then pour into sterilized bottles, cover, and label. Store in the refrigerator for up to 7 days.

HONEYSUCKLE
SYRUP

1 cup honeysuckle
petals

2 cups boiling water

1 cup superfine sugar

1 tablespoon lemon
juice

1. Place the honeysuckle petals in a glass or china bowl and lightly bruise them to release the fragrance. Pour the boiling water onto the petals, cover the bowl, and set it aside for 4 hours.

2. Strain the petals through a nylon strainer, pressing them against the sides to extract as much flavor as possible.

3. Pour the flavored liquid into a pan, add the sugar and lemon juice, and stir over low heat until the sugar has dissolved. Increase the heat, bring the mixture to a boil, and boil for 10–15 minutes, until a light syrupy consistency is reached.

4. Cool slightly, pour into sterilized bottles, cover, and label. Let the syrup cool, then store in a refrigerator for up to 7 days.

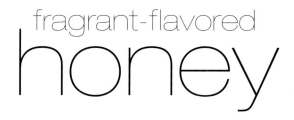

fragrant-flavored
honey

*Imbue the honey of your choice
with the heady fragrance of edible garden
flowers and herbs, for a natural and life-
enhancing sweet treat. Evergreen herbs, such
as rosemary and bay, make an ideal choice for
flavoring honey to create a unique,
homemade gift at Christmas.*

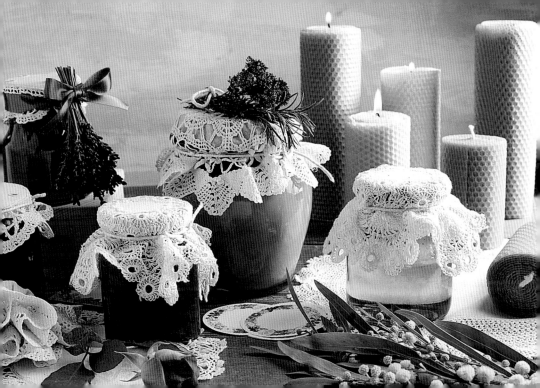

Scented and Citrus Honey

about 6 small sprays of herbs, such as rosemary, lavender, marjoram, or bay, or 3–4 tablespoons scented edible flower petals (see page 372)

1 long strip orange peel

1 tablespoon orange juice

2 pounds clear honey

1. Place all the ingredients in a flameproof jar, cover it, and stand it in a pan of cold water almost to the top. Bring the water to a boil, remove the pan from the heat, and leave it to cool.

2. Leave the honey to steep for 7 days, then gently reheat it and strain into a jar.

Rose Petal Honey

Serve this delicately scented honey spread on toast or muffins, or drizzled over waffles or pancakes.

4 cups scented rose petals

2 pounds clear honey

1. Wash and dry the rose petals if necessary and shred them coarsely in a blender or food processor.

2. Gently heat the honey until it melts, pour it over the rose petals, and process for 2–3 seconds.

3. Pour the honey into clean jars, cover with screw-on lids, then decorate the covers with pieces of lace or decorative fabric and ribbon.

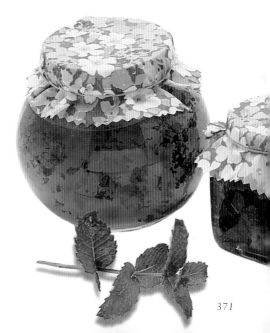

apple & flower jellies

Delight the spirit as well as the tastebuds with this jelly preserve suffused with the scents of fragrant edible flowers.

Choose from carnations, honeysuckle, jasmine, lavender, lilac, orange blossom, scented roses, and violets for a delectable taste experience.

2 pounds cooking apples
juice of 2 lemons
4¹/2 cups water
4 tablespoons dried edible flowers or petals or 8 tablespoons fresh flowers or petals
about 1¹/2 pounds sugar

1. Put the apples into a large pan with the lemon juice and water. Add half the flowers or petals and bring slowly to a boil. Boil gently for 20–30 minutes, until the apples have collapsed.

2. Wring out a cotton, cheesecloth or traditional jelly bag in hot water and suspend it over a large bowl. Spoon in the fruit and liquid and leave to drain, undisturbed, for several hours. Do not squeeze the bag, since this will make the jelly cloudy.

3. Measure the strained fruit juice and return it to the pan. Add 1 pound sugar to each 2½ cups juice. Add the remaining flowers or petals, tied in a piece of cheesecloth. Stir over low heat until the sugar dissolves, then increase the heat and boil rapidly for 10 minutes, or until setting point is reached.

4. Remove the cheesecloth bag, pour the jelly into clean, warm jars, cover, and label. Store in a cool, dark place.

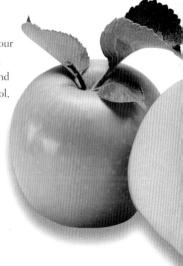

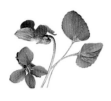

violet
meringues

*These deliciously scented meringues can
be sandwiched together with whipped cream.
Add a little violet-scented liqueur, such as
Strega, to the cream filling for a special-
occasion confection. You can also decorate the
meringues with sprigs of fragrant herbs.*

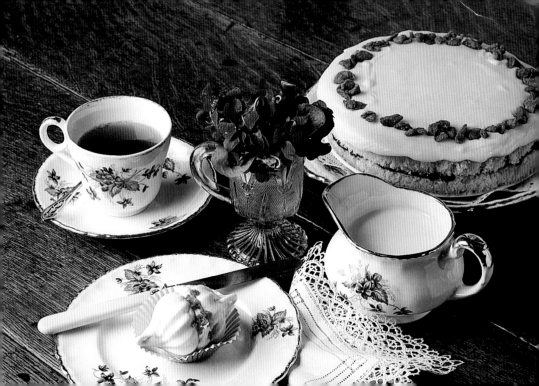

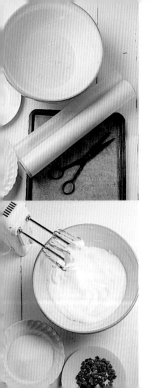

3 *egg whites*
¼ *cup sugar*
4 *tablespoons candied*
   violets
purple food coloring
   (optional)
⅔ *cup whipping cream*
2 *tablespoons powdered*
   sugar (optional)

Makes 10 meringues

1. Line a cookie sheet with nonstick baking paper. Preheat the oven to 275 degrees F.

2. Put egg whites in a large bowl that is free of grease. Whisk them until they form stiff peaks.

3. Whisk in the sugar, 1 tablespoon at a time.

Fold in the candied violets and coloring, if using. Take 2 tablespoons and shape the mixture into small ovals. Transfer these to the cookie sheet. Bake about 1 hour, then turn off the heat and leave to cool in the oven 1 hour. After an hour, wedge the oven door open with the handle of a wooden spoon and leave the meringues until they are completed cooled, about another hour. Remove them from the oven. Whip the cream until stiff with powdered sugar, if you like, and sandwich the meringues together using the cream filling.

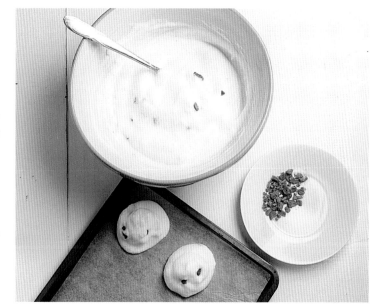

lavender
ice cream

Lavender makes a distinctive scented flavoring for desserts. It is especially good with ice cream. If necessary, you can substitute dried lavender flowers for fresh ones, but if you do, remember to halve the quantity—the flavor of lavender is as powerful as rosemary.

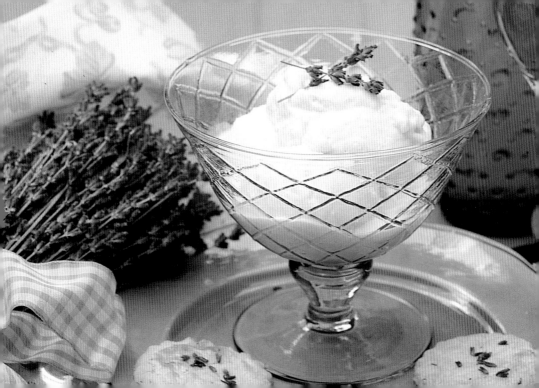

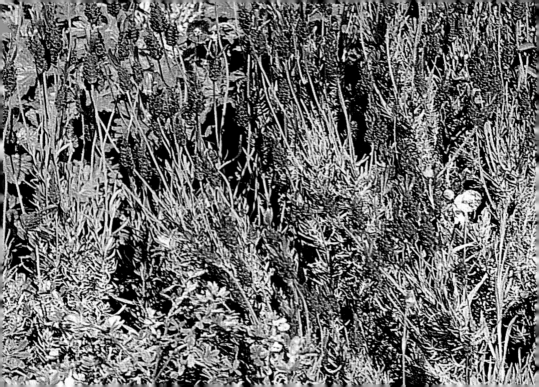

6 sprigs lavender flowers
1 egg
⅔ cup milk
3 tablespoons sugar
½ teaspoon vanilla
  extract
⅔ cup heavy cream

Serves 4

1. Strip the lavender flowers from their stems. Beat the egg. Heat the milk and sugar together with the lavender flowers, and let it infuse for 20 minutes. Pour the infused milk onto the egg, stirring constantly. Return the mixture to the pan and reheat, stirring all the time until it thickens.

2. Strain into a bowl and add the vanilla extract. Allow the mixture to cool, then half whip the cream and fold it in. Spoon into an ice-cream maker or freeze in a container in the freezer, stirring it thoroughly with a fork after about 30 minutes before freezing until it is solid.

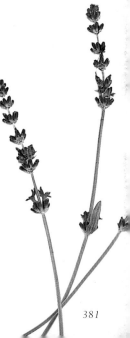

*R*osewater, a distillation of rose petals that has a highly perfumed flavor, has been widely used in Middle-Eastern cooking for centuries. Often combined with almonds or pistachio nuts and cinnamon, it is used in rich, extremely sweet pastries, such as the famous baklava from Greece. Rosewater is also used to flavor desserts in Indian cuisine, notably kulfi, an Indian ice cream.

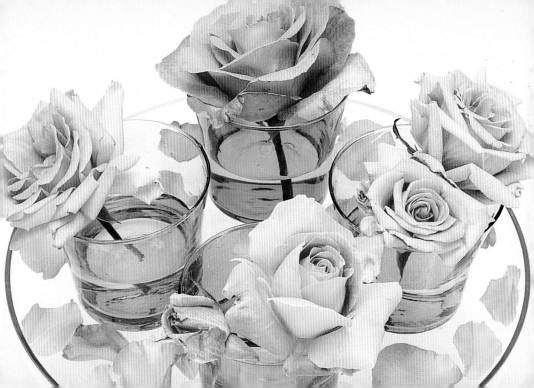

rose-
flavored treats

*The rich perfume of the rose is
another fragrant flavoring that is perfect
for sweet dishes. Add it to your favorite
ice cream recipe or use it in a sweet
soufflé. Check that the roses have not
been sprayed with any chemicals.*

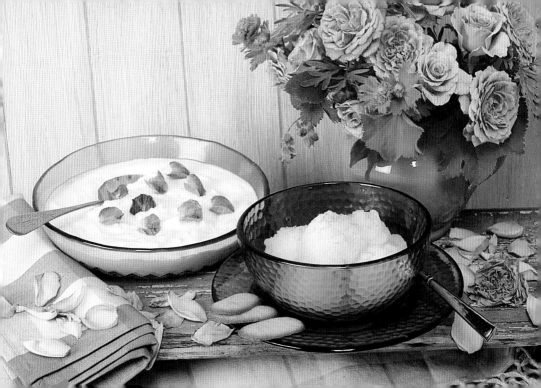

ROSE-PETAL SHERBET

1/2 cup superfine
  sugar
2 cups water
grated rind and juice of
  2 lemons
3/4 pound scented rose
  petals
2 teaspoons rosewater
1 egg white

Serves 4

1. Put the sugar, water, and grated lemon rind in a saucepan. Boil briskly, stirring, until the sugar has completely dissolved, then simmer for 6 minutes.

2. Remove from the heat, add the rose petals, and cool. Strain into a bowl, and add the lemon juice and rosewater. Put the mixture into a shallow tray to freeze for 2 hours until mushy.

3. Decant the mixture into a bowl. Whisk the egg white stiffly and fold it in.

4. Return the mixture to the freezer and refreeze completely. Serve in individual bowls.

ROSE-PETAL SYLLABUB

a handful of scented rose petals
3/4 cup medium-sweet white wine
1 1/4 cups heavy cream
juice of 1/2 lemon
2 egg whites
1/2 cup rose-scented sugar

1. Infuse the rose petals overnight in the wine, then drain off the wine and reserve. Whip the cream in a bowl. Whisk the egg whites stiffly and fold in the sugar, then fold into the wine with the cream.

2. Pour into glasses and chill. Serve decorated with rose petals.

To make rose-scented sugar, mix about 1/4 cup scented rose petals with 1 cup superfine sugar and place in a container with a lid. Store in a warm place for 1–2 weeks, shaking occasionally to distribute the petals in the sugar. Sift the sugar to remove the petals and store in an airtight container.

sweet
geranium
& rose layer cake

This spectacular cake, redolent with sumptuous summer scents, makes an ideal centerpiece for a celebration. Use any red berries to contrast well with the creamy filling and light sponge layers. Dust the surface with powdered sugar and decorate with clusters of frosted berries and geranium leaves.

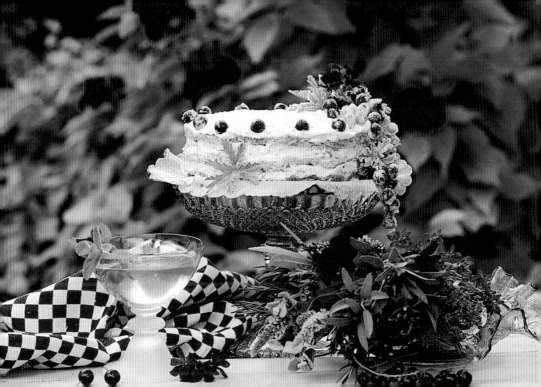

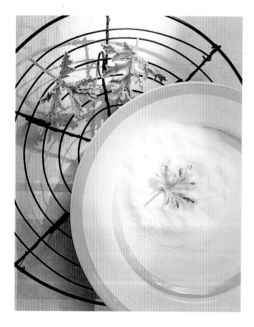

For the cake mixture:
4 eggs
³/4 cup sifted powdered
sugar
³/4 cup all-purpose flour
2 tablespoons cornstarch
¹/2 teaspoon baking
powder
5 rose-scented geranium
leaves, minced

Serves 6–8

For the filling:
2 cups whipping cream
6 tablespoons sifted
powdered sugar
10 pink rose petals,
finely chopped
¹/2 cup berries
(raspberries, blueberries,
cranberries, or
loganberries)
*Extra frosted whole
berries and leaves, to
decorate*

1. Preheat the oven to 350 degrees F. Separate the eggs and put the yolks into a large bowl with the powdered sugar. Whisk until light and fluffy and pale in color.

2. In a separate bowl, whisk the egg whites until stiff, then fold into the yolk mixture.

3. Sift the flour, cornstarch, and baking powder together and add the geranium leaves. Gently fold the flour into the egg mixture.

4. Grease an 8-inch springform pan and line the base with nonstick baking paper. Spoon the mixture into the pan and bake in the center of the preheated oven about 25 minutes, or until the cake is well risen and lightly browned. Unmold and cool on a wire rack. When completely cold, slice the cake into 3 layers.

5. To make the filling, whip the cream until stiff. Fold in half the powdered sugar and the rose petals, then the berries. Spread one half of the filling over the bottom layer, lay the middle layer over it, and spread with the rest of the filling. Place the top layer on the cake and decorate with the rest of the confectioner's sugar sifted over the cake, and the berries and leaves. Chill until required.

at-a-glance guide to

TOP OILS FOR MIXING
chamomile
geranium
jasmine
lavender
neroli
sandalwood
ylang ylang

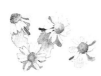

TOP BATH OILS
chamomile
frankincense
geranium
lavender
lemon
neroli
peppermint
ylang ylang

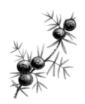

TOP THERAPEUTIC OILS
(body)
bergamot
chamomile
cypress
frankincense
lavender
myrrh
rose
tea tree

TOP THERAPEUTIC OILS
(face)
chamomile
juniper
lemongrass
orange

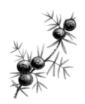

TOP OILS FOR INHALATION
chamomile
eucalyptus
frankincense
lavender
myrrh
peppermint

essential oils

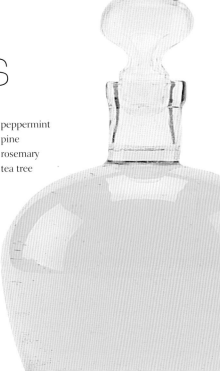

Top Oils for Room Scenting
bergamot
eucalyptus
geranium
jasmine
lavender
neroli
peppermint
sandalwood
ylang ylang

Top Household Oils
cedarwood
eucalyptus
geranium
lavender
lime
peppermint
pine

Top Oils for Hot Poultices
bay
clary sage
cypress
eucalyptus
galbanum
ginger
juniper
lavender
lemon
lemongrass
lime
petitgrain
peppermint
pine
rosemary
tea tree

TOP OILS FOR
COLD COMPRESSES
bergamot
cedarwood
chamomile
clary sage
eucalyptus
geranium
lavender
neroli
patchouli
rose
tea tree
violet

TOP OILS FOR A
THERAPEUTIC
MASSAGE
chamomile
clary sage
eucalyptus
peppermint
rosemary
sandalwood

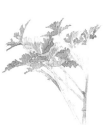

TOP OILS FOR
A RELAXING
MASSAGE
eucalyptus
frankincense
orange
petitgrain
jasmine
lavender
neroli
rose
ylang ylang

TOP OILS FOR AN
INVIGORATING
MASSAGE
bergamot
lavender
lemon
orange
peppermint
petitgrain

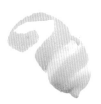

TOP OILS FOR DEPRESSION
bergamot
clary sage
frankincense
geranium
jasmine
lavender
myrrh
neroli
rose
sandalwood
ylang ylang

TOP OILS FOR CHILDREN
chamomile
lavender
tea tree

OILS UNSUITABLE FOR HOME USE
cinnamon
clove
hyssop
sage

OILS TO AVOID DURING PREGNANCY
basil
clove
cinnamon
fennel
hyssop
juniper
marjoram
myrrh
peppermint
rosemary
sage
white thyme

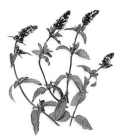
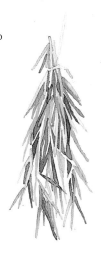

Index

acknowledgments

The Authors

- Gill Tree, Director of Essentials for Health, school of massage pp. 148–73, 176–85, 188–201, 204–13
- Jane Newdick, well-known gardening and cookery author pp. 232, 234–7, 242–5, 272–6, 282–91, 294–9, 300–3, 320–1, 348–52, 356–8, 374–7, 383, 388–91
- Linda Doeser, author of The Fragrant Art of Aromatherapy (Colour Library Books, 1995) pp. 18–20, 26, 145, 214–15, 392–3
- David Squire, renowned gardening author and specialist in plant folklore pp. 10–14, 21–2, 308–13, 316–19, 330, 332–43
- Pamela Westland, widely published cookery and craft author pp. 258–61, 264–6, 364–73
- Hazel Evans, accomplished writer on herbal crafts pp. 222–9, 246, 248–55, 268–9, 280–1, 322–5, 360–1, 378–81, 384–7

Illustrators

- Nicola Gregory pp. 9, 49, 51, 53, 59, 63, 67–8, 74, 79, 81, 99, 115, 127–8, 131, 143, 349, 392-5
- Vana Haggerty pp. 229, 250–1, 255, 325

Picture Credits

- Neil Sutherland pp. 6, 24, 37–9, 91, 139, 145, 187, 235, 305, 311, 315–17, 323–4, 330–4, 336, 339, 340–1, 343, 354, 357, 375, 380, 383
- Di Lewis pp. 29, 35, 41, 71, 95, 123, 129, 203, 216, 231, 233, 236–7, 242–3, 244–5, 262, 273–5, 279, 283, 285, 289–91, 295, 297–8, 301–3, 321, 346–8, 350–1, 353, 356, 359, 363, 376, 377, 389–90
- Nelson Hargreaves pp. 257–61, 265, 267, 278, 365, 369
- Peter Pugh-Cooke pp. 48, 75, 85, 101, 103, 121, 135, 146–7, 152–3, 158, 162–3, 165, 166–73, 176–85, 188–200, 204, 206–13
- Gloria Nicol pp. 4, 83, 133, 218, 221, 223–4, 227, 246–7, 249, 268–9, 280, 313, 319, 361, 379, 385
- Richard Paines pp. 33, 293
- Digital Vision Limited pp. 2–3, 8, 16–17, 73, 306, 309, 329

American Adaptation
Maggi McCormick

Index
Chris Bernstein